UNBREA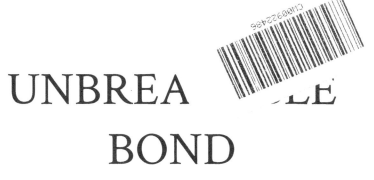BLE
BOND

A HEARTWARMING STORY OF CARING FOR A
LOVED ONE

Adam Sibley

TeamSibley Publishing

I spent four years caring for my mum when she developed dementia and I promised her that I would write a book about our experiences to help others going through the same thing.

This book is dedicated to my mum, June Sophia Sibley, who died in January 2013, when she was 54 and I was 28.

—Adam Sibley 2014

Thanks

This book is a book for the people and made possible by the people. That you have it in your hand is due almost entirely to the following people who got behind it and supported it with their time, energy, skills and finances.

To cover the costs of publishing this book in print form a crowd-funder campaign was started and in less than a month over 20 people had helped reach the target. So before you embark upon reading my story please join with me in thanking the people who made it possible to share it with you:

Alan & Francesca March of Alan March Sport Ltd
Alex Mclean
Mark Sanders
Tim & Michelle Parkman
Julia Gorski
Kalle Hogh
John Shaw
Kizzy Wroath
Sheryll Murray
Ginette Nye

Dolores McCormack
Triona Murphy
Robert Davidson
Kym Wain
Dean Seddon
Mikki Walker
Jane Hoblack
Steven Kandes
Steven Beattie
Lindsey Brittlebank
Gwyneth McLoughlin
Barry Matthews
Lacshan Manoskanthan
Kevin Marriott

All of you made this possible.

CHAPTER ONE

What is it to be a Son?

I made my life about being the best son to my parents I could possibly be. I don't know if I ever achieved it or came anywhere close. I don't think I even knew what went in to being a good son but it didn't stop me trying. My parents were my world: I put them above everyone and everything else. I would spend more time with my parents than anyone else and I always couldn't wait to spend more time with them.

When I was at school I couldn't wait to be back home again. I would go home for lunch. Outside of school in the evening or weekends I would want my parents to go everywhere with me and if they ever had to go anywhere I would always ask to go with them. I hated being left at home or going places without them. I would enjoy the car rides, the watching TV – just any little thing I could.

I would always find ways in which I could help my parents, whether it was doing things around the house or helping with shopping. There were lots of things I couldn't do but everything I could do, I would — and I would at least try to do something, even if it was probably more of a hindrance than a help.

I put my mum and dad above everyone else; their well-being and happiness was far more important than my own. As long as they were happy I was happy. If they were ill I would want to look after them and help them get better. I would always be so sad if they did get ill. My wish as a child was that I would die before they did. Very morbid, I know, but I would have sacrificed my life for them if it helped them.

I liked buying them cards and gifts on their birthdays, Christmas and anniversaries. But I didn't stop there: anytime I had money in my pocket I would want to buy them something. If I didn't have money I would make them things or give them things that I already had.

I could never be too generous when it came to my parents. I just wanted to show them in any way I could how much they meant to me. Nothing was too much. I always loved giving them presents more than I did getting any myself and they got me some lovely presents over the years.

Now I'm not saying the way I set about being a son was right or wrong, I'm just saying how I was when I was growing up. My one hope has always been that my parents knew how much I loved them and how proud of them I was. I would always boast about my amazing parents to everyone I could and when people came round to our house I think they could see how close we were just by seeing our day to day life and they would be envious of what we had.

As mum would go everywhere with me people would get to know her as 'Adam's mum'. My friends also became friends with my mum and when I went somewhere without her they would always ask where she was. People were always so kind to my mum, involving her in conversation. It must have seemed weird to everyone else as no one else brought their mum with them to things like I did but no one made me or my mum feel uncomfortable about it.

I think the role of son changes at a very rapid rate. You go from being fully dependent on your parents to them being your world, to moving away and starting a family of your own, who then become your world. Sometimes these changes can happen without you realising. I think it is important that regardless of life's changes and the time you spend with your parents that your love for them never changes.

I think one thing that is becoming more apparent and more the norm is that sons and daughters will have to look after their parents in later life. Sadly, however, this isn't something that enough people think about or make plans for. I know its something that nobody wants to think about. You don't want to think of your parents getting ill but it is something that we all need to be prepared for.

Changes in health can happen in an instant and can turn life upside down so if you don't have a plan life can fall apart quite quickly. So it is in your and your parents' best interests to have planned ahead. Don't expect others to do it all for you; this is the moment where you can pay your parents back for everything they have done for you.

You may have to start caring for your parents earlier in life than you expect. You may not have had much of a life yourself and you may be very young. You may not know how to care and have no experience but this isn't a time for dwelling on things or running away, it is a time for facing life head on and standing up to the challenge.

The one thing you need to remember is that regardless of who is caring for whom in your family you are still a son and your parents are still your parents and that never changes. There is no getting away from it and there is no changing it and I would like to be remembered as somebody that never forgot it and was the best son I could be for as long as I could be. To me, this is the mark of what makes a great son.

The life of a son is a life of devotion. There will never be anybody more important than your parents in your life so there will never be a more important job that you get given than the one you were born with and that is being a son or being a daughter. The challenge is: 'can you make your life that life of devotion; can you make your life the life of being the best son or daughter you can possibly be?'

CHAPTER TWO

The Importance of Mums

I don't think there is any person more important in someone's life than a mum. What a mum goes through to bring you in to the world is something that can never be repaid. The amazing thing is that mums don't want or need this 'debt' ever repaid. They do so much but ask for nothing in return. After doing everything to bring you into the world they keep doing more for you and more and more. They never think they have done enough – at least that's my experience.

I think being a parent and being a mum are two different things. A mum is someone who has a relationship with their child, a mum is someone who cares for their child above everything else and would do anything to protect them and to give them the best life possible. This was the story of my mum. My mum was a mum and never just a parent. To my mum we were a blessing and never a burden and even during her battle with dementia she put us first and wanted everything for us. My mum gave everything she had and never asked for anything in return. The only dream my mum ever had was to want our dreams to come true, regardless of how silly or far-fetched they seemed.

My mum never criticized or judged and never asked us to change. She never tried to make us do anything or stop doing anything, she just supported us in every endeavour or pursuit we had. Mum stuck up for us if anyone ever thought badly of us or if we were in trouble and she would always defend us no matter what. If we wanted anything she would help us find a way to get it. These are just some of the many ways in which our mum was a mum to us in every sense of the word.

My mum took a huge interest in anything I was interested in. She would research and ask questions about it and take a look out in the media and would tell me when a programme about that certain thing was on. When I liked a pop star or an actor mum would let me know if they were on a chat show and if I wasn't home she would record it for me. No matter how uncool the music or TV I liked was, she would pretend it was the coolest thing in the world and would have no problem going to a concert or a film with me that I would be embarrassed to ask of my friends to go to.

I think a mum brings something to a child's life that no one else can do and I think people who don't have a proper mother playing a proper mother role in their life are missing out and that it will have an effect on the person they grow up to be. There is a different kind of love and support that a mother can give that is different from the love of a dad. I'm not saying one is more important than the other but a mum is a person we all need in our lives.

My mum was a stay-at-home mum and I know that in many families mums can't afford that. I loved my mum being a stay-at-home mum and I am so thankful that she was as I don't think I would have turned into the person I am today if it wasn't for that happening. My dad went out and worked and was away a lot of the time supporting the family financially so my mum would have to be all things rolled into one, which she did amazingly.

A mum not only has to go through carrying you and giving birth to you, putting her body through an incredible ordeal, but from then on has an almighty list of tasks she has to perform. Not only does she have to bring you up but she also has to manage the house and in some cases to work at a job outside the house as well as to maintain her relationship with your father.

Once a woman has a child she is no longer responsibility-free, no longer can she put herself first or just think about herself. No longer is she free to do whatever she likes. Now all decisions revolve around you and now she has to be careful about how she acts in public as this all now reflects on you and her ability to be a mother. This can be a tricky transition to make and people are not in-built with these abilities and skills. It is a way of life that a mum must pick up as she goes. Being born into this world is a start – giving birth to a child is a life change.

When I was caring for my mum during her battle with dementia she would tell me to go out and do things. She felt so guilty that I was staying in to look after her and not going out. When she needed me the most she would still put me first. She hated being a burden but to me she never was. The relationship I had with my mum was a two-way street: she cared for me as much as I cared for her. I was never going to not put her first in her hour of need. Even when things got bad she would use all her strength to give me a smile and the one phrase she held on to until the very end was "I love you," which she would tell me as often as she possibly could – and every time she did it was the highlight of my day.

Even during my mum's battle with dementia I could see in her eyes and her actions that she still wanted to help me and be the one supporting me. She would try to hide her pain so I didn't witness or feel what she was feeling. When things were going wrong she would tell me not to worry about it. If something went wrong and she realised it wasn't quite right she would try her best not to draw attention to it and change the subject. Mum was my protector from the day I was born to the moment she died; the one thing she never forgot was her role as mum and that I was her son.

My mum was so important to me that I would drop anything to help her, I would give up anything I had for her; my time, my money, my possessions – if it helped mum, I would do it.

My mum had a fun challenge looking after me and my two brothers. And she did the most amazing job of it. She made sure everyone was loved equally and that no one felt like a favourite. My mum did her best every day to spend as much time as she could with all of us and to help all of us to achieve our dreams. When us brothers fell out she wouldn't take sides regardless of who was in the wrong; she would act as mediator and get us back talking again. She made sure we supported each other and kept us together as a family whilst letting us all be individuals in our own right as we were three very different people.

My mum's daily schedule would be based around making life as good and as easy as possible for us boys. When she went to the shops she would always buy us treats and when it came to birthdays and Christmas she would always make sure the same got spent on all of us and that everything was fair. Mum never made us do anything that we didn't want to do or push us into anything. If she could see we liked something she wouldn't let us give up if we failed, she would make things as easy as she could for us and find different ways of attacking things. If you were ever having a bad day she was the one person you wanted to speak to.

If it wasn't for mum's love, support, advice (both emotional and practical) I wouldn't have turned into the person I am today. I will forever be my mum's son and I think that is the proudest thing I can say about myself. My mum makes me who I am and will continue to have an impact on the way I live, the decisions I make and how I feel until the day I die. That is how I can keep her with me and let her know every day that she was beyond important to me.

CHAPTER THREE

Caring

I think caring for someone without the want of pay or reward is the most amazing, selfless and worthwhile thing a person can do with his or her life. Helping someone who is in need or who wants to do something they can't do without help is something that all able-bodied and able-minded people have the ability to do. It's just that in this world not everyone uses that ability. There are so many things that we can do that we take for granted, so many things that we don't even need to think about or strain to do. But for some people these very basic and simple things might be the hardest things to do. I couldn't imagine not being able to do some of the things I take for granted.

Imagine watching other people round you being able to do everything without any help and not being able to join in or do what they do. Imagine the embarrassment or the pain it might cause someone to have to be helped with these most basic of tasks. Imagine how inhumane it must feel and how intolerable it must be. I don't know about anyone else but if I saw that happening I couldn't help but go over and offer my support.

I think that in the British culture we aren't as understanding and accommodating as we should be of people who have disabilities or who need help. Instead of rushing to help or just be nice to them we are instead asking what is wrong with them, pitying them, ignoring them, moving away from them or a million and one other worse things. I think we take our health for granted at times and that many people don't realise how lucky they are to be fit and healthy and not need help from anyone. We are so lucky to live in a world where in many countries the number of fit and healthy people who require no assistance far outnumber those who are not so lucky yet not enough people are helping.

Through the experiences of looking after my mum I became more aware of, and started to think more about, the way we view mental health. I can't stand the way, as a culture, we use the word 'mental' to refer to/insult people with mental disabilities. I can't stand how it is viewed as something to be scared of, with people thinking "don't talk to or go near people displaying symptoms of a mental illness as they are frightening" yet they would talk to someone with any type of physical disability and no one would be scared of them.

In this fast-paced society we seem to have no time or understanding for people with mental illnesses. Many sufferers can't control what they are saying or their behaviour but people choose to distance themselves from them, which is such a crying shame.

You can't judge people with mental illnesses by your own standards. Just because you know what is right and wrong or the accepted process for doing things it doesn't mean someone with a mental illness does. You can't shout at them for doing something wrong or get annoyed with them because they don't know or think they are doing anything wrong. Shouting at them or getting annoyed will only make things a million times worse for you and for them.

If a loved one of yours was battling with mental health problems you would want people to be compassionate to them and you wouldn't want to think of them being ill-treated by others. If you are not with the loved one you are caring for all the time they will interact with people who aren't family on a regular basis. It was so important to me that when I was away from my mum everyone treated her with love. I would panic every time I was away from her, thinking that someone might not be treating mum as nicely and as well as I did or treating mum in a way I wouldn't be happy with.

When caring for my mum I always wanted her to live as close to normal life as I could possibly make it. I wanted her to be able to experience everything that anyone else could. This meant we would go out and about to public places a lot. Being out and about when caring for someone brings with it a lot of challenges, one of which is that you are so focused on being a good carer that you sometimes aren't as aware of what is around you as normal. I was always hoping that people would notice this and make allowances for it. I found that ringing ahead helped, so that places like cafés, shops and tourist places could be ready for our visit.

My main dread when going out with mum was people either staring at us, laughing at us or just not understanding and not making allowances. Even though dementia awareness is on the rise you would be surprised at just how many people couldn't just notice the signs or put two and two together.

On the positive side there were places and people that did help my mum and me when we were out. We never forgot and built up great relationships with the best people and places. We would go back and visit regularly and they would make mum feel like the most important person in the room, going out of their way to make it the best visit possible for her. Some places just aren't set up for being able to handle someone with dementia, which is totally understandable but it just meant that we became very choosy about where we went and frequented the quieter places because when I took mum out I wanted to make sure that I never stressed her out and that she always had a good time.

I think more needs to be done by the government and society to recognise those that give up their time freely to care for others. I think these people save the country a lot of time, resources and money. Without them I think it would put a major strain on the NHS. To give your time and your life to help someone in need is an amazing thing to do. People who do it shouldn't have to live with the stress of having to find money to pay for the basics. When their time being a carer comes to an end more should be done to help get them back on their feet and into work. I bet that if someone cared for a person for, say, 20 years whilst not working and put that on a CV for a job their CV wouldn't be picked against someone with recent paid work experience.

Caring for someone can seem like a daunting prospect especially if you are anything like I was and you don't have any skills or experience to call upon. But I don't think caring is about that; to me caring is about love, patience and selflessness, which are things you can't learn on a job. I think the best carers are those that don't realise that what they are doing is caring and those that don't realise what an amazing job they are doing. I think you can judge your heart on that moment when you are faced with a loved one needing care and what action you take. Do you take responsibility or do you let someone else deal with it and pass the buck?

I think the more the person you are caring for knows you and the more you know about them the better carer you will be. You may be able to get in the highest qualified carer in the world but for your loved one they may be more comfortable with having you care for them. You may not know all the things a professional carer does but no one is going to be able to love your loved one more than you. So when thinking about the caring arrangement for your loved one always think what would be best for them and not you.

I know if I needed care to do things like changing and going to the toilet I would prefer to have a loved one rather than a stranger help me. When a loved one is going through hell I would want to do whatever I could, no matter how big or small, to make the situation as good as it could be.

Don't get me wrong, caring for a loved one is not easy, especially if it is a parent you are looking after as it is quite a reversal of care roles. It can take a lot of getting your head around to understand that you are now looking after someone whose normal role has been looking after you. I have so much admiration for kids up and down the country who have taken on the role of carer from such an early age. There are so many children in the UK that don't get the chance to live a childhood of their own due to looking after a family member and I salute all of them. Giving up playing and going and seeing friends when you are only a kid is the most amazing selflessness.

If you have lived with the person you are caring for all your life it can really change the dynamic of the house. You will probably have to pick up more jobs around the house and your daily routine may be quite drastically changed. Now not only do you have to do more around the house but you also need to factor in extra caring time, which wont leave you as much time as you use to have to do other things. The types of conversation had in the house will change, some people may stop coming and you may have to stop going out. Caring for someone will change every little facet of your life but to me it is so worth it.

It can hurt so much seeing someone who used to be the most physically and mentally agile person go downhill and not be able to do the things they used to be able to do or just be the person they used to be. Disability can really affect the person you are caring for on all levels; their mood and character may change, which will affect the mood of the entire house. It is also hard not to get sad and depressed yourself witnessing the changes first-hand and seeing a person you care for dearly not being able to do all the things they used to do.

Caring for someone you love is the most challenging thing you can do in my opinion and will test you to your physical, mental and emotional limits. It will test your ability to adapt, your problem-solving skills, your ability to smile and your ability to carry on even in the darkest situations. But it is all worth it to bring just the smallest shred of comfort to someone you love or bring a smile to their face. In good health or bad health, that has always been my aim. My aims never changed but the ways I achieved them did and the longer the condition went on the more creative I had to become but I always found a way to achieve them.

Remember that age doesn't make a good carer. Someone can be amazing at caring for someone at eight and someone can be great at 80. Don't underestimate the internal power and ability to care for others. You can be the most intelligent person in the world and not know how to care; intelligence has nothing to do with caring. The ability to care is based on your internal strength and your ability to deal with situations around you. Never let anyone make you think that you can't do it. Be wise enough to learn and take advice, as well as asking for support when you need it, but don't let others put you off.

Don't let other people be sorry for you or sad for you because you are caring for someone. Those emotions can rub off on to you and affect you. On the flipside, if you're not sad about it don't let other people be sad on your behalf. You don't need to be sad about caring. Even though you are sad for the loved one you are caring for you don't need to be sorry about caring. You are allowed to enjoy it; there is nothing wrong with that.

CHAPTER FOUR

Love

There is nothing more important in life than love. Love can make you do things you never thought possible. Love can make you feel emotions and things you never thought possible. Love is the thing that gives you a reason and purpose in life. Love is power and love can give you energy. Love can, however, at times make us take rash decisions or fail to think clearly. So be warned: love is a strong emotion that we need to learn to use in the right way.

There is no greater gift in life than love; it is the best thing to receive and it is the best thing to feel. I think the feeling of love can be one of the most comforting and happiest things in the world. Love makes you smile, it makes you feel warm and it can make you feel better. It can take you away from the harsh realities of life and can make you forget bad things for a moment. It can give you hope when something seems hopeless and for all of these reasons I think when caring for someone the most important thing to do is to love them.

When you are having a bad day or things are going wrong it is important to remember that you are loved and that you love others. Never lose sight of the love you have for the one you care for and the love they have for you. Never take it for granted and remember to put that above everything else. Always make sure the one you are caring for

17

knows that you love them at every opportunity. Sometimes the person you are caring for may not be able to express or show their love for you but I am sure that if they could they would be shouting it from the rooftops.

Love can make you do incredible things; it can make you do things you never thought possible. Things that seemed impossible can become possible with love. It can enable you make the hardest of sacrifices and make these sacrifices gleefully, with no bitterness in your heart. Love will make you the best carer and make you feel good about what you are doing.

There was no one I loved more on earth than my mum and I would have done anything for her and I tried my best to do that every day. Love isn't just about telling someone you love them, giving them a hug or a kiss, although these are really nice ways of showing love. To me a stronger show of love is through your actions: what you are willing to do for the one you love and the lengths you are willing to go. Love is about being selfless and doing everything with the right heart.

Love can make you smile, love can make you sad, love can make you angry and love can make you laugh. There is nothing wrong with feeling and expressing all these things but when you are caring for your loved one you can show them only the positive sides of the emotions. The one you are caring for will feel scared enough or bad enough for what you have to do for them so they don't need to be made to feel any worse.

If you see someone you love going through a bad situation you are going to feel angry. When I found out about my mum I was angry but if you are angry because of your love it shows how deep your love is. The best thing to do is to let it out but do it out of sight and out of earshot of the one you are caring for. Don't be afraid to cry, either. It's good to let it out but do it out of sight of the one you are caring for. Strong emotions make you a great carer; without that emotional connection you wouldn't do what you do.

You want to produce an atmosphere of love in the house. When other people come in the house you want them to show love, to love the one you are caring for and to love what they are doing. If you can do all these things you will be providing an amazing place to care for your loved one.

There may not be a cure for the condition your loved one is suffering with, you may not be able to change their life expectancy but with love you can make every day the best it can be. That is your job as a carer and if you can do that you and your loved one can look back at life and know you made the best of it.

CHAPTER FIVE

Isolated

Regardless of how many friends or family you have around you, you can still feel like the most isolated person in the world when caring for a loved one. Caring for a loved one is so all-consuming that you can easily sometimes not recognize, realise or feel the love and support from them. You know they are all around you but it is so easy to have the philosophy of 'it's me against the world' or that no one else cares or knows what you are going through. When all of your thoughts, emotional energy and time are wrapped up in one person you don't have time or emotional space to think and care about others as much.

There is so much advice and support out there but even reading every leaflet, being in every care group or regularly seeing specialists, that isolated feeling is still hard to shake. You just think to yourself that they don't really care or that they can just go home at the end of the night and live an ordinary life and forget about you.

When caring for someone you always think you know best and that no one knows the situation like you do. This can make you quite resistant to help or support, as you are worried people won't handle the situation properly or in the way you would want them to. This can lead to you deliberately isolating yourself from others. Sometimes it's just a case of being a private and proud person and you just don't want people putting their noses into your business. In other cases isolating yourself can be a way of just switching off the real world because you can't cope with everything that is happening. It could be that you want to live in denial of the current situation or you don't want to spend your time thinking about the world and its problems. Sometimes it just hurts to go out and see people not affected by what you are going through, not knowing about it and living happy lives when that is something you can't be a part of. There are many reasons why sometimes we isolate ourselves deliberately from others.

You start thinking that others can't possibly care for your situation. Why would someone else care? Why would they want to stop and take the time to help? When someone offers to help or do something you just brush it off as you think they won't make good on their promise. You know it's not other people's problem but you still want them to help you and when they don't it can hurt. Sometimes you just wish people wouldn't promise to help if they aren't going to as it builds up your hopes and when they don't follow through it tarnishes your opinion of that person.

When we are going through something so bad it is so hard to comprehend that someone else could be going through it too. You don't think it is possible and you don't want to think that it could be possible. Sometimes you isolate yourself because you don't want to experience any more bad things or have to deal with any other bad news, so by isolating yourself it limits the number of bad things that you think can happen to you.

Geographical isolation can be hard to deal with. If you live in a remote or rural area it can make life more challenging. It can make getting to the doctors, hospital or the shops tricky and sometimes shops will not deliver to you if you live in a very remote area. Living in a remote area can stop people from coming to visit you. It also makes it more of an effort to go anywhere to get things or do things, not to mention the time and cost it adds to the simplest of tasks. If you don't have a car of your own you will feel even more isolated, making it impossible to do many things yourself.

The form of isolation that hurts the most, though, is the isolation you feel when you go out and about. When people see you are caring for someone with a disability people will deliberately avoid eye contact, walk in the opposite direction, cross the street and try to close down any conversation you may start with them. People seem to view people with a disability as people to avoid or be scared of. In the world we live in more and more people are likely to suffer from a major illness or disability in their lifetime yet we are nowhere near as kind and compassionate as we should be. This, more than anything, can make you feel like you are on your own without a friend or a friendly face in the entire world. When I went out with mum I took her out so she could interact with different people and different things. But sadly I found that most people couldn't even take a few minutes out of their day to interact with us or make conversation. My mum loved people and loved making friends so it made it so hard for me to see it happening in front of my eyes. Not only were they isolating mum but me as well.

No matter what statistics tell you, you always think you are the only ones going through it and that you question why it is you that has to go through it. It is very hard to control how isolated you feel. Sometimes you can feel isolated by an event, sometimes by circumstances and sometimes by emotion. Isolation can take many forms and happen for many reasons. I think the healthiest thing to do is to stay as engaged in the big world and with people around you as possible. They may not understand what you are going through or be able to support you but I find many people are great listeners and can just help break up the day a bit rather than just shutting yourself away from the world outside your door.

CHAPTER SIX

Hiding

It's a fact that more of us may have to care for someone in the future. Yet caring for a loved one seems to be something that very few people contemplate, which only makes it harder for everyone involved. Let's not sweep under the carpet the current problems we have with care. Let's celebrate those who care for others. Let's make these people our heroes. Let's make these people respected and looked up to in communities. It is the carers who will have a huge impact on the community, making sure those that are unwell live as full and happy lives as possible and don't become a burden on the community.

Let's live in communities that look after each other. Let's not be the ones to just call someone crazy if they are acting differently; let's be the ones that love them and get them help. Let's not be too scared. Let's remember that people who need caring for are people just like you and me. By doing this you make communities that more people are happy to live in and give fewer people the chance to moan, complain, be scared of or make fun of people so they can use their time and energy in a positive way. We are all inhabitants of this world and although we may not be related it should be our responsibility to help each other. You might have lots of friends and family; if you do, you have to know that is such a privileged position and that not everyone does. Some people have nobody and it is good to recognise these people when they come along and be that somebody for them. Some people who are all by themselves need that help from someone; everyone else might have passed them by but don't let that be you.

Everybody is born entitled to the best life possible so let's start behaving in a way to enable that. If someone can't live that best life by themselves – help them; it's that simple. This is a real difference that everyone can help make happen very easily. If you keep helping people you will change lives. It may not happen today, it may not happen tomorrow but believe you me, some day it will. Once you have changed someone's life in this way you will have something to be proud of and it will enable you later in life to look back on it with a smile. Just remember that as well as helping others to this 'best life' you need to make sure that you get yourself that best life too.

We have freedom of speech in this country but we rarely use it for the right reasons. Never be put off talking about a subject or feel that you can't bring it up. By not telling someone what is happening to a loved one you are hiding. If you think something is wrong you need to speak up because it is that action that might save their life. Don't be afraid to talk to others about caring and illness. Don't let it be a subject we can't talk about because you talking about it will help others to talk about it, which will have a snowball effect and before too long everyone will be empowered to talk about it. If everyone is talking about it then it keeps it in the public conscious and in the public eye which is where subject of care needs to be.

Don't hide from yourself and don't hide from life. The more you hide the less able you are to deal with problems, then the more problems will mount and grow until one day you can't handle it any more. Don't hide from your friends and don't hide from the world. Be confident to let the world know who you are and what you are going through. Although not perfect, I think the country becomes more accepting of differences every day. Nobody that hides away can change the world.

CHAPTER SEVEN

Guilt

There wasn't a day that went by when I didn't feel guilty. I would feel guilty about the biggest and the littlest things. The biggest thing I would feel guilty about was the fact that my mum had to put up with this terrible illness but I got to get up and enjoy a healthy life. Mum had given her whole life for others, never spending a penny or second on herself or for herself – and what did she get for it? An incurable, intolerable and horrendous illness. Finally, in a time of life when my two brothers and I had grown into adults and my mum's job was done and she was free to put herself first, the first signs of the illness started to show, ruining any chance of enjoyment mum had to look forward to in life. My biggest wish was that I could change places with my mum and take the illness for her. She had given everything for me and I hadn't had the chance to do anything for mum. I had just started my journey into adulthood so with the onset of the illness I knew this was going to be the only chance I had to help mum and I just found it beyond cruel that I couldn't trade places with her.

Regardless of what I did, I always thought I hadn't done enough and could have done more. If I ever got annoyed, cross or angry whilst looking after mum it would eat me up inside and I would feel like the worst person in the world. I so wanted mum to beat the illness and was every day trying so hard to keep mum's cognitive function and her ability to do things going that when mum couldn't do something I would feel myself getting frustrated inside and kept trying to get her to do it.

I felt that I was doing something wrong and I knew the more abilities mum lost the closer we came to not being able to look after her at home, which scared the life out of me. I wanted to keep mum at home forever and didn't want to admit to myself what was happening and what was going to happen, I would grip on to any small success I would have with mum and that's why I tried so hard every day as I needed that glimmer of hope to hang on to.

Mum was a very proud person and used to like knowing facts on everything so I loved giving mum a sense of achievement every day. Seeing her smile when she worked out a puzzle or beat me at Scrabble was worth a million pounds. I would always praise every achievement and loved seeing mum feel good about herself. But I would always feel guilty about pushing mum too hard when she had days when she wasn't doing as well at the puzzles and challenges I set her.

The moments in the day I felt most guilty were the moments when I wasn't with mum. During the early stages of mum's condition I would feel guilty about going to work and leaving her at home by herself, to the point where I wanted to quit work to become a full time carer. Luckily, as mum's condition progressed we got support and people came in to sit with her during the day so I was able to feel less guilty on that side. This wasn't the end of my guilt, though, as I still thought it should be me that was doing the caring and I always wondered what was going on at home when I was at work. Mum loved me and couldn't comprehend that I had to work. She must have felt like I was abandoning her every day, which was a thought that wouldn't leave me until I got home from work and was able to give her a hug. I would go in to work early so I could get home early and as soon as I left work I would rush as fast as I could to get home. I am so thankful for everything that the company I worked for did for me, how flexible they were, so that I was able to help mum as much as I could whilst still keeping a job.

I am heavily involved in volunteering through coaching five teams at Liskeard Girls' FC, of which I am the Chairman. I was also the Treasurer for Truro Hospital Radio as I am so passionate about these two causes. Both these endeavours required a lot of my time and whenever I was doing work for either of them I would always feel guilty about not spending that time with mum. When I didn't get involved in events to do with these organisations I always felt guilty about letting them down. I would try and do as much work as possible whilst mum was asleep but much of it had to be done during the day so I would rush to and from events so that I could get home to be with mum. This also involved leaving meetings early and leaving other people to pack things up so I could get home.

With mum, work, volunteering and family it meant that my friends got a raw deal and were often pushed to the back. All I wanted to do was spend time with mum so I was closed off from a lot of close relationships because I didn't have the time spare to invest. My oldest friends understood but it meant I couldn't make new friends. It also meant that when people invited me to things I had to make up excuses as to why I couldn't go for the three years of mum's illness. Whilst I was making excuses I had to then hear stories at work or between my friends of things they had been up to or hear about them on Facebook.

There were so many things I wanted to do with friends and hearing about things they were doing when I couldn't tag along on was difficult. After a while people stopped inviting me as I was always making up excuses. I'm sure some people thought I was making up excuses because I didn't want to go but that couldn't be further from the truth.

Out of respect for my family and mum, no one outside my closest friends knew what was happening at home. Then when I was wishing I could do things with friends I would feel guilty for thinking like that, as seeing friends would take me away from seeing mum.

I would feel guilty for telling my closest friends what was happening with mum. It was like I was betraying her and I would then feel guilty for lying to people about mum and not telling them.

I put every last bit of effort, time, emotion and thoughts into mum so it meant I wasn't there for the rest of my family like I should have been. I wasn't the best brother to my two older brothers and wasn't the son to dad that I needed to be. I didn't spend enough time with the rest of my family and wasn't there enough for them when they needed me. I didn't ask them how they were often enough and I didn't help them through a very difficult time. I would put mum first and I always thought I knew best when it came to mum and that I should be the one to do things for her or with her. My actions stopped the rest of my family having the time they should have had with mum, for which I will always feel guilty. I feel guilty that I didn't let them spend 'alone time' with mum because even if they were around I still wanted to stay with mum as well. I felt guilty for not letting more people in to help mum but I always thought I knew best when maybe I should have got more support.

I didn't research the condition of dementia enough as I was spending all my time with mum. I didn't question what doctors had said. I just went along with what was going on. I didn't push enough for mum to be sent to see more qualified specialists in the field or to have her case reviewed. I didn't research enough about medications or alternative therapies that were out there. If I had known more about the illness I could have provided better care and got mum better treatment that might have changed the outcome. I just got so fixated with mum's day-to-day well-being I didn't look at the big picture. When you are in the middle of a situation it is so hard to take a step back and look at something objectively. No matter how many people tell you that you did everything you could, you always feel like you could have and should have done more. I am guilty of being in this club but I just can't help feeling that way. Nothing was ever too much for my mum and I could never do enough for her. I just wanted to do all I could all the time for mum and that is how I spent my life with mum.

CHAPTER EIGHT

Anger

Anger is an emotion that takes up a lot of your life when something like what happened to my mum happens. I wasn't sure who I was angry at but I was angry that someone as amazing as my mum could be diagnosed with something so horrible. The thing with dementia is that it has no respect for character, personality, intelligence, importance or impact someone has had on the world. You could be the greatest or worst person in the world and you can still get it. I just found myself asking why someone who has given everything for everyone else should have to go through this.

I was angry that there was no cure for dementia. With the money that gets put into medicine and with all the advances in medicine and technology, how could we not have a cure? Why isn't there a way to beat it? How can a brain just shut down? These were just some questions going through my head. Nothing seemed to make sense and the less sense it made the angrier about it I would get.

I would find myself getting angry with other people around me, complaining about the most trivial things. I would think to myself 'You don't know how lucky you are.' I hadn't told anyone about mum so how were they to know. And bad things are only relative to what else is happening in your life. But for some reason it would still annoy the life out of me. I would hate going on Facebook and reading posts about other people having bad days. I didn't own pain and I had no right to cast judgement on others but I just couldn't stop myself. Being angry at others seemed to be a way of not being angry at what was happening to my mum, which hurt too much for me to cope with so it was a phase I had to go through.

I would get angry when looking at photos of friends going out and doing things, seeing other people leading happy, healthy lives and going out and having a good time. I wished that could be me so badly at times. I resented them so much for it; for having a good time without me, and I was angry I couldn't be a part of it. People were moving on without me and they were building memories and strengthening their friendships. I would get angry about people not asking me if I wanted to go out and do something any more because I kept having to make up excuses.

I would get angry about how easy other people's lives were and how carefree they were. They never had to be anywhere at a certain time or not do something because of other commitments like me. They could go away somewhere or move for a job opportunity. They could travel with work or friends. They could have a bit of independence, get a place of their own, devote all their time to a hobby or another half; they had no restraints and no restrictions. Sometimes I just needed a break, physically and emotionally just to be normal for one day, with no stresses or strains, is what I craved. But I never wanted to leave mum and always hated it when I had to, so that just remained a dream because I loved mum too much to have a day away from her.

I would get angry about friends who didn't come and see my mum even though they knew about her condition. I always wanted mum to be surrounded by friends and love so I would hate it when that wasn't happening. The one thing that I would hate the most, though, is when people promised they were going to come over but never made good on their promise. At times there just didn't seem to be the support that I thought should be there. It just felt as though my family and I had been abandoned on our own to deal with everything. Mum was no one's responsibility except ours but I just expected others to help us out a bit too much, which was what caused the anger.

I felt so angry about the time that it would take to get things done for mum – to arrange support, attend appointments etc. The paperwork and the *bureaucracy* would drive me round the bend. There just seemed to be so much wasted; time trying to get somewhere but sometimes getting nowhere, when all of this time I could have been spending it with mum. There was information overload about everything to do with dementia but it made it very hard to decide which was the right path for mum or to know what support mum should or shouldn't have.

One main source of anger was that looking around at my friends and colleagues and seeing how many of them had fit and healthy parents I seemed to be in the minority. No one else had to care for someone in their family. Some of them even barely saw their mum or dad, and some wouldn't have a nice word to say about their parents. I loved my parents and lived with them yet I didn't have what most others seemed to have and take for granted. I would have given anything to be in their shoes and have a fit and healthy mum. Why should anyone in their twenties have to be a carer for a family member?

All this anger was illogical and I would find myself getting angry about being angry, if that makes any sense. I had my mum and dad so what more could I want? My mum wasn't angry with anyone or anything. My mum didn't want me to be angry and all the time I spent being angry wasn't helping me be the best son I could be to my mum. What did I have to be angry about? I was fit and healthy and I had a mum who loved me.

CHAPTER NINE

Hopelessness

When caring for someone with an incurable illness that is progressive you can be gripped by the feeling of hopelessness. When this happens you can feel like giving up and just become frozen and do nothing. When nothing you do seems to help or make any difference, when the harder you try the more things seem to go wrong, you keep asking yourself 'what's the point of doing something if you can't see the results you want from it?'

When you feel hopeless it is hard to be positive and it's hard not to show this hopeless emotion outwardly. Then when you start showing in your actions and character that you are feeling hopeless that can catch on like wildfire to other people around you. The more people that catch on to how you feel the more the atmosphere will change and the more negative life will become for you and the one you are caring for. People around you may not know how to speak to you and may avoid you if you are feeling hopeless, as they don't want that feeling to rub off on them and for them to act and feel like you do. Positive and happy people like to be around like-minded people, so if you want these people in your life you need to be like them.

The one person you can't afford your hopelessness to rub off on is the one you are caring for. If the one you are caring for starts feeling hopeless it can speed up their deterioration. Now I know it is not advised to bottle things up and to try and lead a life of something you are not but it is important to choose the right times and the right people to let these emotions out at or to.

You can't go back and change things and you don't want to live a life full of regrets. That is why it is important not to let the hopelessness grip you and stop you from trying. Regardless of what the outcome is or looks to be, if you try every day to do everything you can to help and make life as good as possible you will have very few regrets later in life.

There is nothing wrong with feeling hopeless and there is no weakness in it. It is a very normal and human reaction when faced with a situation in life like this. It is just very important that you don't feel bad about it and try to disguise the fact that you are feeling like this. It is good to have someone outside of your caring situation that you can trust that you can go and talk to about it and let it out.

If there is someone else in your caring situation that you think is feeling that hopelessness, talk to them about it and support them. Tell them about how you feel and try your best to make them feel as good as you possibly can. Encourage them to speak to people outside of your caring situation, such as other friends and relatives. Let them know they have done nothing wrong. Don't be scared to talk to them about it. Don't let them just continue to slip into this feeling and don't let their attitude effect the atmosphere in the house. Even if someone is older or higher up in the family hierarchy, you have to say something. Saying nothing is helping no one and is the coward's way. Talking about these things is scary and you have to be brave to talk about them but it is the best thing you will ever do. Your relative or your friend may be waiting for you to ask them and may want that opportunity to talk about it but be pretending to be happy or not saying anything because they don't want to bring others down or look weak.

Regardless of how you feel, you have the strength to be a leader. If no one else is stepping up, it's up to you to do it. The more open and honest approach you have to those around you the better you will be able to manage everyone's emotions and feelings. The better everyone is feeling and coping the better you will all be able to care for your loved one, as everyone needs support, including you. Know when to put your happy face on, know when to open your ears and know when to talk. Do all those things at the right times and you can't go far wrong.

CHAPTER TEN

Friendship

Friendships are one of the hardest things to keep going when you are caring for a loved one. You make friends with people before you know you are going to have to care for someone and the caring situation could have been something you never expected. The friends you make never think you will have to care for someone either. When you make friends you make them your priority and you make as much time for them as you possibly can. Little or no forward planning is needed. You just knock on your friend's door or give them a ring and you hang out without giving it a second thought.

A friendship takes time and investment to grow; it doesn't just happen. A friendship needs effort and work; the more you put into a friendship the better they get. Friendships need all this on a constant basis. The moment you stop doing all this even the best or strongest friendship can unravel, as it is not about what you have done in the past it is about what you have done recently.

The more friendships you have the more time out of the day it will take. Most people like more than one friend and most have a group, and with that group you will quickly find yourself getting in to a weekly routine of hanging out and doing things together. Nothing beats that feeling of a friend ringing you up or texting you to invite you to do something.

41

With some friendships not even a day will go by without you seeing your friend.

The situation with your friends can quickly change when you start looking after a loved one. At the drop of a hat your priorities change. Suddenly, instead of planning life around your friends, you have to start planning around caring for your loved one. It is when this starts happening that you find out who your important and biggest friends are – if any. Your friendships go from being two-way streets to your friends having to do much more of the work and it will test how much they really want to keep the friendship going.

When caring for a loved one, time and energy are two things you don't have for anyone else. When your friends keep inviting you to do things and you keep saying no, the number of invitations will start to dwindle until they don't bother inviting you to anything at all. When a friend perceives they are doing a lot of work and not getting much in the way of friendship in return they may move on.

A key battle to fight can be whether to tell your friends about what is going on in your life. Some people, when caring for others, don't like letting others in, so may choose not to tell them what is going on. If that is the path they choose, it is near-on impossible to maintain friendships, as your friends will have no clue why you suddenly stopped calling, going out or making an effort for them. Some people want to say something but can't out of respect for the privacy of the loved one they are caring for. This is a personal choice but I feel if these friends are important to you and you want to keep them in your life you have to let them in a little way. You don't have to go into specifics or tell them everything but you have to give them something so they understand and can make adjustments and accommodate you and your needs.

I think if you do tell your friends anything about what is going on you have to let them know straight away what you can and can't offer them in the way of friendship so everyone knows where they stand from the start. It will save anyone getting annoyed later. You have to expect that some may not think the effort is worthwhile to keep the friendship going and you have to expect that they will find other things to fill their time with if you aren't around as much. It's hard but try not to get offended by your friends' actions. When caring for a loved one you may have little time for your friends so don't waste that time talking through or creating problems. Just go out there and enjoy it and use it for that much-needed respite.

If you have a big group of friends you may need to just choose a small group to stay in touch with. Don't think this is a bad thing. It will be impossible to keep all the friendships going and if you try, you will fail, believe me. So choose the people that matter the most, the ones you truly can't live without, and work on those relationships. It is better to have a couple of strong relationships than a host of weak ones. Don't feel bad for the friends that you lose; they will have other friends and find new ones. You won't have the emotional energy and strength to worry for others, so sometimes you just have to let them go and move on. There is nothing wrong with it.

With the friends you do keep, you have to be prepared to be yourself around them, warts and all. When caring for someone you will have to keep a brave face on around the house but when you have that time out of the situation you need a break from doing that, so don't feel you have to keep it up in front of your friends. Your true friends will understand that you need that time with them where you don't have to pretend, so never feel you have to pretend for your friends or to be strong. If you have given them enough information about what is happening they should be prepared for this.

There never seems to be a right time to tell your friends what is happening. Telling your friends you are caring for a loved one can be hard to get into a conversation. There also may be times when you know your friends are going through stuff, so you don't want to add to their load or because you know the news will affect them you don't want to bum them out with the news that depresses you the most. When your friends are happy or you are happy laughing with your friends you don't want to dampen the mood, so you don't want to tell them during these times, either.

A big problem that comes is 'how many friends do you tell'; would you feel bad telling one and not another? If you want the news kept to a close circle of people, do you want to burden them with a secret and can you trust them with it? It's not a pleasant feeling when someone comes to you that you haven't told saying they are sorry or are thinking of you. When this happens you don't know which of your friends to trust and it makes you angry that someone has done it. When you deliberately tell only a select group of people you do it because you don't want the whole world to know. A really bad time is also when a friend finds out you have told some people but not them as that can make them annoyed or hurt if they thought they were a close friend and should have been. With friends you just have to hope that they accept that the reasons for your actions are because of your situation and not because of them. When caring for a loved one there is very little you can control and the world at the best of times can seem very out of control.

Try not to spend time with or make friends that are a lot of hard work. Generally, 'down' people will take up a lot of your time. When you are going through hard times you need positive people around you that are there for you and won't ask for much in return; people who won't get annoyed and just accept you for who you are. Never worry about what a friend is doing when they aren't with you or what your caring situation is doing for the friendship. Just make the best of the time you do spend together –that would be my advice to anyone currently going through those problems. Friendships should add to and improve your life, not take away from it and make you miserable. Don't take on other people's moods and problems. Just try and be the best friend you can in the time you have. Never feel you have to act in any particular way around a friend. If being happy and upbeat works for you, do that; if being melancholy helps you, do that. No one who is a true friend would judge you for the way you act.

Don't have high expectations of your friends; don't expect them to do things for you and to help you. The more you expect from them the more disappointed you will be. If you don't expect anything and they give you something it will mean the world and then you don't have to worry about any disappointment. This situation will be new for them as well as you so they may not have all the answers any more than you do. It is all a learning experience for you as well your friends.

If a friend wants to help, try to find a way that they can. When caring for a loved one you may think you don't want anyone else helping you. There maybe things you want to do yourself for privacy and dignity reasons so avoid having help with these. Caring for someone can also involve a lot of routine activities so although you may not be able to involve friends in a direct caring role they could help you pick up things or sort things out. You may think you know best when it comes to caring and you may not want anyone else caring for your loved one but just having someone with you when you are caring can make it a more pleasant experience and can make you feel less isolated. This is a way you can get someone to help without burdening them, which worked well for me. If you are always asking a friend or always burdening them they may start getting annoyed and distance themselves from you

It's not just your friendships that are important. The friendships of the loved one you are looking after are equally important. With my mum I always encouraged people she knew to come over and spend time with her or I would take mum to their houses. I think seeing familiar faces and having friends really helped my mum and lightened up her days. Morale and positive energy are important to the loved one you are caring for regardless of what they are suffering from and I think friend-ship can help provide this for them.

If you are close with your loved one it may be that you have mutual friends. Spending time with these people is important as it means the friend can support both of you at the same time and you can spend time with them whilst caring. Never forget that to be a great carer *you* need support, too. I was lucky enough to be friends with many of my mum's friends, which made the caring process so much easier on everyone. Never underestimate the power of friendship.

CHAPTER ELEVEN

Working

When you are trying to balance work and caring for a family member it can get very tricky. It's not your workplace's responsibility to be flexible to your caring needs and the demands of your role as a carer can change on a daily basis. I can see why many people are forced to or choose to give up work in order to care, as the stress of trying to do both is quite unbearable at times. If push came to shove I would always choose leaving my job to be able to care for a family member but I understand why some people's financial situation would mean they wouldn't be able to do the same thing. If you are the only one earning money leaving work could mean risking losing the house or not being able to afford to pay bills, which could have a major negative impact on the care you are able to give the person you are caring for. Although we have the NHS, caring for someone can be quite expensive at times, especially providing for any special requirements necessary to care for the person properly.

The other option some people go for is part-time work as this enables you to work and care for someone without the workload being too high. But again the money earned working part time might not be enough to cover bills so may not be an option for some. I think it is important for the carer, especially when caring for a family member, to get a bit of respite on a weekly basis and to have something outside the house to focus on so a part-time job could be a great way of achieving this. Spending time outside the house can refresh you. Speaking to different people and working can also just make you feel a bit normal again, if only for the briefest of periods. When you live with the person you are caring for it is a 24-hour responsibility so those small breaks are vital. This is, of course, possible only if you have someone to care for your family member when you aren't there.

A problem when a loved one needs care is that they can't work any more and if they used to work and contribute to the paying of bills it will leave a big financial hole to fill. This may mean you need to look for a different job, take on more than one job or do more hours. You may be stuck in a horrible position of not wanting to work but not being able to stop work. You may also have to give up on pursuing your own personal career goals to get a job that fits best around your caring situation. You may find yourself doing a job you hate but thinking it is worth it because it is the best job to help with being the best carer you can be.

Getting carers in whilst you are out working can be expensive and defeat the financial objective of working. So to keep working you may need to call on friends and family members to help you. The only problem with this arrangement is that if a friend or family member lets you down your boss will still expect you at work so it could lead to you getting into trouble at work or leave no one to care for your family member. It is also a big ask for friends and other family members to help as they more likely than not won't have any training or know how to deal with the situation. This may mean a lack of a decent standard of care for your family member or a strain being put on your friendship with the person you ask to help, so you need to be careful when doing this.

The other thing you can do is speak to your local council and see if you qualify for professional carers to come in and their cost be covered. It can be very strange having someone you don't know come in to your house and work but it can also be beneficial having a trained profession-al to learn from and give your family member a great level of care with-out it putting stress on you or a friend. You have to be mindful of how your family member will react to someone new and whether it is in their best interests. As a family member no one will be able to show the person you are caring for more love but that doesn't mean you are cut out for caring or doing the right thing. Although it's hard, it is some-times in their best interests to bring professional support in.

When caring for someone it is important you stay as fit and healthy as possible, mentally and physically. Make sure you are getting rest and are physically capable of doing everything you need to do. When you are tired, stressed or unable to care how you want to it can affect the way you care for someone. Without knowing it or meaning to you can do something wrong or snap, which would not be in your family member's best interests.

It is important not to take your stress from your home life to work – easier said than done, I know. When you are at work you are being paid to do a job and what is happening behind the scenes shouldn't come into it. It is especially important to remain professional and in control if you haven't told anyone at work about your situation because if you do act a bit erratically they won't know why. If you have told people what is going on they may be more lenient with you but don't forget that every-one at some point in their life goes through personal or family problems, so there will be people around you in your workplace who may be struggling as well.

Remember never to take your problems out on the people you work with or burden them with your problems. If they care and take an interest, share how you're feeling or what is happening but as a carer the caring is down to you and is your responsibility. The colleague may have been asking just to be nice so don't expect them always to be there for you and them to care like you do. It is important not to be too dependent on others, as they will have their own lives to lead and their own problems.

One of the hardest situations is if you are caring for someone and run your own business. When you run your own business you have a lot of responsibilities to keep it going, keep it generating money, functioning within the law, and in many cases the responsibility of the staff that work for you. At least when you work for a company there isn't as much pressure on you and the organisation won't fall apart if you don't go in.

Continuing to run your own business will be especially hard if you used to run it with the person you are caring for. Running the business without them may take an emotional strain and a strain on your time if you are now doing the work of two people. The problems will be compounded if you run the business from home but at least if you do you can balance work and caring a bit better. Another hard situation would be if you used to work with the person you care for in another organisation because going to work won't be the same without them and people will always be asking after your loved one.

When you are working it means you can't always drop everything to attend to an emergency at home. You can ask to and some companies may let you but you then may need to make the time up, lose pay or get yourself in trouble. If you are looking to climb the company ladder and you keep on having to take time off at the last minute it won't look good to your employer. If you need to take time off to go and sort things out at home and your company don't let you, you can start getting bitter towards the company or have to run the risk of being disciplined for disobeying orders and leaving the job.

Outside of the caring that was going on I always wanted to be at home as much as I could so I could be around mum. I knew one day we would lose mum to a care home so I just wanted to enjoy every moment I could in mum's company. When she was going through something so awful I just wanted to be there to hold her hand and make her smile.

When I was at work it was hard to concentrate on the job as I was always thinking about mum and trying to leave as early as possible every day to get back to see her. When you have all that happening at home it affects your enjoyment at work and your levels of concentration, which means you start making mistakes at work or do a slapdash job, which your employer will eventually see. If your employer does see it then it can hamper your chances of promotion and could lead you into disciplinary procedures.

If you are out of work and find yourself needing to work to support the person you are caring for it can be quite hard. Unlike other people, you may not just be able to take any job: you will need a job that fits around your caring and helps your current situation. This will limit what you can apply for and I know it shouldn't but it may put people off employing you if they think you won't be committed to the company and may need lots of time off. When you start in a company you have to pay your dues and you don't get many favours. Normally, it takes you putting in several years of hard work and loyalty to get special treatment or favours in your company. Being a carer, you might have been out of work for a while as well, which may not look good on the CV and if your need for work is desperate it may take a while before you find a job and get paid from that job.

Use work for whatever purpose you need it: for respite, for a change of scenery, for escape, for something to challenge you, for a chance to talk to other people or for a chance to make money. Whatever your reason, find what it is and remember that every time you go to work as it will make work far more bearable. The one thing you don't want to do is go to work and hate it then go back home to care in a bad mood as that isn't going to help anyone. Try not to get agitated at work and go home in a worse mood than you were in when you went to work. If you use work correctly it can really help you be a fantastic carer to the loved one you are caring for. It is OK for a period of your life when you are caring to put your personal needs over those of the company you work for and to be less focused on your career.

I think if you are to keep on working and caring at the same time you need to be organised, let your company and colleagues know what is going on and have procedures in place in case there is an emergency. This could mean enlisting the help of friends and neighbours to support you. Don't forget that although you are the one caring for someone you need support too if you want to be the best carer you can be, which should be the number one aim.

CHAPTER TWELVE

Routine

When caring for someone your life will become a life of routine. It seems like the best way to care for people is through routine. To make sure everything happens and nothing gets forgotten, it is routine that makes this possible. It is so important not to forget one single aspect of a loved one's care, so that routine can become vital. Routine is also important if you have a myriad of people working to care for your loved one, so that if someone else takes over they know what has and hasn't been done.

When making life easy for your loved one, routine is important. If you do have many people caring for your loved one it is less stressful if your loved one knows when they are coming. Someone dropping in out of the blue can sometimes have a really negative effect on the loved one you are caring for.

I'm not saying spend your whole life in routine as from time to time you need to break it (with things like day trips and holidays) just to enhance your life and that of the person you are caring for. Doing the same routine day in day out can be quite draining and may not stimulate the one you are caring for. You want to make your loved one's life as rich and exciting as possible so look at your routines and schedules and think what are the best moments to be spontaneous, when are the best times to mix things up and have a bit of a change.

The person you care for may have good days and bad days, so you have to have the ability to adapt routines accordingly. When someone is having a bad day they may need a higher level of support and when they are having a good day it may be a great time to do one of those breakaway from routine ideas. It is sometimes frustrating when you plan in advance something special for your loved one to do and when the time comes they are having a bad day. Just remember this isn't their fault and is the problem with forward planning when caring for someone. If this happens, see if you can change your plan for another day. If you can't do that just try to make the best of the situation and look at ways you can adapt the event for everyone to get something out of it. If you go into a day with a negative attitude it isn't going to help those around you.

CHAPTER THIRTEEN

Time Management

To be a good carer, time management is one skill you are going to have to learn. When caring, it will seem like you need more hours in a day but try as you might it is impossible to get them so you have to learn how to make the most of the hours you *do* have instead. Time management is about maximizing your time whilst doing it in a way that is the least stressful and tiring. There is an art to it. Not everyone has the ability and people have different philosophies on it but it is something very much worth learning.

Time management helps keep your life in order and organised. Without time management you don't know if you can fit things in or what you have coming up on the horizon. If you don't know how much free time you have you may say 'no' to doing something you could have fitted in or you might say 'yes' to doing something when you have no time to do it.

If you decide to go down the route of working and caring, time management will be crucial to the care you can give your loved one and crucial to your own mental, emotional and physical fitness. I think the key thing to remember when it comes to time management is that caring is about quality time, not the quantity of time. It's one thing making sure you are there for your loved one as many hours as possible in a day but if that means the time spent caring is not quality time (with you being stressed, tired or worrying about where you have to be next) then the quantity of time is worthless.

Time is precious, so use it wisely. The first thing you have to do is make sure you are getting enough sleep or rest during a day because if you don't start with this you may find that although you are able to spend lots of time with your loved one in the short-term you will soon burn out and damage your own health, so long term you will be setting yourself up for a fail. When I was caring for my mum sleeping used to be one of my favourite times of the day. Sleeping was the only time when I could switch off from the hurt I was feeling inside and was the only time to escape the stress and the worry as well as all the bad and evil things in this world. So not only was sleep helping me function during the day, it was providing mental and emotional relief from the things going around in my head. Depending on the situation of the loved one you are caring for, sleeping maybe difficult but you need to try to find a way somehow to make sure you get as much rest as humanly possible or else you will be no help to anyone.

The next thing to do is to work out how much time you have left in the day outside of work to care for your loved one. When do you leave for work and when do you get back? Could you change how you get to and from work? Could you change your hours slightly to avoid rush hour? Could you go home during your lunch break? These are all important questions that need to be answered. I know it is hard with some jobs but it is good to know in advance what times you will be leaving for work and getting home as it makes planning the rest of your day a lot easier. If you have children you need to drop off or pick up from school can you work out a way that will not impact on the time you have to leave and the time you get home?

Then comes time for prioritising, decision-making and sacrificing. If you have a lot of things on your plate and are involved in a lot of things outside work like I was, you will be in for some tough decisions. When caring for someone they become your priority and there is no way you can successfully balance caring, work and a busy life outside of work. For some people time outside of work is spent socialising, volunteering, doing projects or just relaxing but after working and caring there is going to be very little time for this. My advice would be to pick one thing you like to do and try to do a little bit of that when you can when you are not working or caring.

When I started to help care for my mum I was involved in several organisations as a volunteer, which I was never going to be able to keep up. So I made the hard decision to leave three of these organisations, all of which I cared passionately for and enjoyed volunteering for. But it was an easy decision to make as it meant I would be able to spend more time caring for my mum. I was never one for spending lots of time relaxing at home doing very little. I get bored if I am sitting down for too long so I never had to give up any of that but if you are a more re-laxed person than me cutting into your relaxing time could be a huge sacrifice. I also wasn't one for doing projects outside of work. I have friends that do anything from music to DIY projects. I know that people get so much pleasure from doing things like this so it must be a huge part of their life and may be hard to give up but giving your loved one the best care possible means sacrifices will have to be made.

The huge sacrifice I had to make was my social life. I loved going out with friends and doing things with them. I hated being by my self; I always loved company. When I started caring for my mum I had very little time for socialising, so friendships got strained and became distant. I lost some friends and lost the opportunity to make new friends but I just saw time spent with friends as time not achieving much when I was trying to care for my mum, work full time and be heavily involved in two big voluntary organisations.

My motto throughout this whole experience was that it is better to do a few things brilliantly than do a lot of things awfully. The thinner you spread yourself, the worse job you are going to make of the things you are doing. And the time you spend doing them will be for nothing if you aren't doing a good job of them. So choose realistically what you can do and what you want to do, focus on those areas and give it your everything. Remember, your priority is your loved one, not an organisation, not a project or a social life.

Don't show misguided loyalty to your workplace or an organisation you volunteer for. It is so easy to get in the mindset of thinking these people need you and that they wouldn't be able to function without you. Another important thing to remember is that by leaving you are not letting them down and they won't hate you forever, they will understand. After you leave, someone else will come in and the machine will keep on working. By you leaving an organisation it frees up a space for someone else to come in or for someone else to stand up and take on your workload. Just be up front and honest with the place of work or organisation and they will understand. Don't just keep doing it because you are scared of leaving. If you leave an organisation and it does fall to the ground that's not your fault either. If that were to happen that would be the fault of the organisation for making it too reliant on you. It wouldn't be your fault. If it does fall to the ground it's not your responsibility. If you can't bear to leave completely just ask for a sabbatical, explain the situation and say you can't put a timeline on it but when situations change you will be back.

When caring for a loved one you have to be strong and you have to make tough decisions. It may not be easy but in the long term you will thank yourself for it because it is so easy to waste weeks, months and years trying to keep it all going. Remember that every day is critical when caring for a loved one, so you need to act fast.

A good time management tool is to think of all the daily tasks you do and think if you can do them with the loved one you are caring for? Consider everything, from the mundane things like cleaning, washing etc. to the eating, shopping and so forth. The more things you can involve your loved one in the better. Doing this can help you keep on top of things and not let things fall behind or the house become a state. Depending on the condition of your loved one, you may be limited to what you can do but even if it is just one or two small things it will help. You should try to minimize the time you have to spend away from your loved one doing the daily tasks so it doesn't cut into your caring but also then you won't be spending time when you are not caring doing these tasks when you should be relaxing or having some time to yourself. Great time management is about making as much time for caring and as much time for relaxing as possible. Involving the loved one you are caring for in day-to-day tasks like this could also do wonders for their morale. It could show them that they can be useful, still contribute and do things they used to. It may give them some value and feeling of self-worth. Doing day-to-day tasks may also be a good stimulant or therapy to cope with whatever illness they are fighting. That's ultimate time management, when you are getting things done but also providing an activity that helps the person you are caring for at the same time.

If you really want to get in to the nitty-gritty of time management you can. Start by looking at every task you do in the day and the order you do them in. If you re-ordered them, would it create more free time? Is there a way you could change each process to make it quicker? You may also like to think of the layout of your house and where things are kept. Is there any way you could move things to make them quicker to find or quicker to access? Knowing where everything is in the house can save you a lot of time running around like a headless chicken trying to find things you have lost. Are there any gadgets and gizmos that you can buy to speed up regular tasks? I know you always see these type of things on home shopping channels but it does no harm to have a look and see if there is anything out there that can help and speed things up. If it would save you only a few seconds here and there I wouldn't bother but if you find it frees up some serious time in a day or over a week, I would think about doing it and making the changes.

To free up your time you also need to think 'is there anything I do that I could get someone else to do?' If you have money, you could pay a gardener, a cleaner etc. Or instead of trying to fix the plumbing yourself you call an expert. If you haven't got money, are there friends, neighbours or family who would help, even if it were the smallest task of posting a letter or getting some shopping for you? Never be afraid to ask for help or outsource anything that isn't about the direct care of your loved one.

No one can control how much time they have on this earth but we can control what we do with it. Whilst we have time left life is about making the most of it and not letting any go to waste. Don't dwell on things or put things off. Don't clutter your life up with things that don't matter. Don't do things just for the sake of doing them. Don't look back wishing you had given up something sooner than you did. Decide what is best for you and your loved one and do it to the best of your ability.

CHAPTER FOURTEEN

Balancing Act

When caring for a family member life can seem like one long balancing act. You spend a lot of your time questioning whether you have got the balance right and sometimes it may seem impossible to balance all the things you have going on. In these circumstances it is important to remember that it isn't always possible in life to balance things 100%.

The fewer things you have in your life, the easier it is to balance them. Simplification is the easiest way to balance things. First you need to get rid of anything that isn't essential or important and then put what you have left in order of priority. At no point in life is everything going to be of equal importance. In these situations you have to be brutally honest with yourself and ask yourself what are truly the most important things. Think to yourself what are the things you could drop without anyone being affected. Think what jobs or things can be put off or done later; think what things in your life can be passed on to others.

Sometimes it is going to feel like you're scrambling to find the balancing point but try as you might you can't find it. If this is you, don't worry and don't panic. You will go through seasons where life isn't in balance for a reason. Sometimes life tests you to see how you can cope when life isn't balanced. Sometimes life is meant to be unbalanced because you should be favouring stuff that you wouldn't normally over everything else. Sometimes the only way to deal with a situation is to focus your energy in one or two areas for a time.

If you are working, raising a family and/or volunteering whilst you are caring for someone, life will feel like you are running from one thing to the next with no time to stop. Life will be about timings and planning. It's not only you that may have to make sacrifices but others around you might have to as well to help you balance everything you have going on. To do the balancing act you may need to rely on the help and/or support of others to make it work. Sometimes it is impossible to do it yourself or it may be possible but at the cost of putting too much unneeded stress and strain on yourself that may affect you later down the line. Accepting or asking for help from others is not weakness, it is great strength and may be the only way to make the balancing act of life work, so don't feel bad for doing so. If by doing this you can free up more time to look after your loved one or take away some stress, which means you can give your loved one better quality time, then it will be so worth it.

Doing the balancing act can be a daily battle, which may change from day to day with new challenges. The important thing to remember with every decision is that it is all about putting the ones you are caring for and your loved ones first whilst not forgetting about yourself. The moment you lose sight of this will be the moment it all falls apart. What you are doing may seem strange to others; others may not understand and some people may be annoyed about it but never let that affect your thinking and just go out every day to make sure it is the best day for the ones you care for and love.

The important thing is to make decisions that put the one you are caring for first despite their being so many people that want your time or think that you should make them a priority. In my life I have always been a 'yes' person. As soon as anyone asked me to do anything I couldn't help but say 'yes,' even if I didn't know how I was going to fit it in or how I was going to do it. You need to learn it is OK to say 'no' or 'sorry' I'm busy.' You can't be something to everyone but you can be everything to the person you care for and that is what is most important.

When you have your life in balance there is no guarantee that it is going to be in balance tomorrow or remain in balance for a long time. Every day different things and unexpected things will happen, especially when you are caring for someone, that will throw your balance off. The key is not to add more to your plate and always be ready to reorganise, as it might mean tomorrow's changes actually make the balancing act easier.

Don't beat yourself up when you get it wrong because, trust me, you will. Life is about decisions and as humans we don't always make the right ones. You can start thinking to yourself that you didn't put that person first there or you should have put that person first then. Sometimes you are forced into making quick decisions but the key is never be afraid to change your decisions if it is going to make balancing everything easier.

Never expect others to know the decisions you have had to make or why you had to make them. Many people won't understand how difficult it is to balance things when caring for someone. When you put first someone else that depends on you it changes your way of thinking and what is important to you. The only way people will understand it is if they have been through something similar in their own life. Never waste your time trying to make others understand. It may be frustrating or hurt you sometimes when people don't understand what you are going through but just telling them isn't going to give them a real appreciation of what you are going through.

All the juggling and balancing may seem like the hardest thing ever – and to the point of being impossible at times – but it is so worth it when you get to spend time caring for the one you love. Giving up things may seem like sacrifices, having to reorganise your life might be hard, and you may start questioning why you are doing it, but all of this goes away when you are with the one you are caring for. Personally, I think it feels better to be sad for sacrificing something whilst spending time with the loved one you care for than going out and doing something and sacrificing time with the love one you care for to do it. There is nothing worse than making sacrifices to go out and do something and then not being able to enjoy something you should be enjoying or normally enjoy because you are thinking you should be somewhere else. When you have a loved one going through so much pain it is hard to find a reason to enjoy anything. The only thing I could enjoy was bringing a smile to my mum's face when she was going through the hardest pain in life.

If you try to balance on one foot for a long time it is hard not to fall over. All it would take is getting nudged or a strong gust of wind to knock you over. The best way to balance is with both feet on the ground. If you try to balance something the best way to do it is to have lots of supports under it covering all angles. The same approach needs to be taken to perform the balancing act of you caring for someone. The more support you have and the more people you have propping you up the more in balance you will be. You may not be able to spend the same amount of time doing things you used to do but in this phase of your life you have to think less about time and more about proportion. Have you got everything in your life in proportion and in the right proportions? That is the question you need to ask yourself. Is it fair that you spend more time doing this than that and vice versa?

One thing to remember is that even though you put the person you care for first you need to remain a balanced and healthy person yourself. So you need to factor in some respite time and, most of all, you need to balance your sleep. The only way you can be the best carer you can be is by being fit physically, mentally and emotionally. This mean sleeping right, eating right and getting the emotional support that you need. If you have no time to cook, try to get someone in to help you, and if you need rest ask someone to come and help you. One thing life has taught me is that time is about quality more than quantity and this is a balance that needs to be struck to get the most quality hours of caring possible.

CHAPTER FIFTEEN

Hobbies

Before you start caring for a loved one you have lots of free time on your hands. Most people spend their evenings and weekends doing the things they like. A lot of people will have an interest or something they like to do, from playing football to going to a stitching group. You may not go to an organised group or be part of a team. What you do might be an individual pursuit or just something you like to do on an ad hoc basis. Many people use these activities to let off steam from the day and for some people it's what they get the most joy out of doing. They may hate their job or things going on at home but the thing they choose to do as their hobby is what they look forward to in the day.

For me, having a hobby is very important and I think can help you deal with life and your day. Having a hobby gives you something to look forward to; something that is just for you and something that can keep you physically, mentally and emotionally healthy. I think that everyone should have one and everyone should find time to do one.

When caring for a loved one it is easy to run away from all your hobbies and devote all your time and energy to your loved one. You want to do what's best by your loved one and if you do two or three hobbies you couldn't prioritise one over the others, so they all go. This can feel like the right and selfless thing to do. I really enjoy volunteering in my spare time and I was working for several organisations but it was just impossible to keep doing that and care for mum at the same time. I could have just walked away from them all but instead I asked myself which ones could I work around caring for mum? I prioritised the list and managed to cut it down to two and found ways of making it so I could do both without affecting the level of care I gave my mum in a negative way.

Thankfully, the organisations were very kind in the way they dealt with me. Those I had to stop volunteering for were very understanding and the ones I stayed with allowed me to work my volunteering around caring for my mum. Never be scared to say 'no' to people and don't think you have to explain yourself, either.

When I was caring for my mum a lot of my hobbies would become more house-orientated, like watching TV or going on the Internet. Yes, I know they aren't the best hobbies but they were a way of relaxing and escaping whilst still being in the house if mum needed me and during the times I was caring for mum it was something we could do together. I would find programmes we both liked to watch on TV and I would find things on the Internet she would be interested in, or in my personal time I would search the Internet for information and support on dementia.

Don't feel like your hobbies have to be a regular commitment. It doesn't have to be something you do daily, weekly or monthly. It could just be something you do sporadically when you feel like it or can fit it in. Sometimes by doing something sporadically it means more and you get more of a buzz out of doing it as it is more of a treat than a routine thing.

You will get a lot of people that want to do things with you but never be afraid to go and do a hobby on your own. Alone time for yourself is important so if you want that time to do something by yourself it can help to go somewhere where you know nobody and can be invisible for a while without the fear of someone giving you sympathy or asking how things are. If alone time is important for you then see if you can link it in with a hobby, something that gives you that respite you need and may help you physically, mentally or emotionally. A hobby shouldn't be there just for something to do to meet people and get support; it should be an outlet for you and something you enjoy doing; something that maybe restores a bit of normality for even the smallest fractions of time during your day.

Before my mum went rapidly downhill I would think of hobbies outdoors that we could do together. We found places we liked to walk, as mum loved the outdoors; places to have a hot drink, as mum loved hot chocolate, and places with animals as mum loved animals. We went to zoos, wildlife parks, safari parks; you name it we went there. I got an allotment so mum could come out and sit on the allotment whilst I worked it and maintained it, which during the summer was great fun.

Just be careful not to get too engrossed in your hobbies and have them take over your life. Sometimes it's hard not to get drawn completely into the world of your hobby as it is so much fun and such an escape but remember you are doing a hobby for a bit of 'your' time, not to have it dominate your life. Think 'how much time do I want to and how much time can I devote to it' and use that time to the full – no more, no less. If you feel yourself getting drawn in and spending more time doing a hobby than you should, don't be afraid to rein it in again, as this will be easier the less immersed you are in it.

CHAPTER SIXTEEN

Adapt and Overcome

When you care for a loved one in your own home, adapting and overcoming will be a way of life. Most of your life will be spent trying to do these two things to get things done, to make things safe and to care in the best possible way. The normal house wasn't built with caring for people in mind. The house is laid out and furnished in a way to make it look good or to fit in with your usual life routine. When buying and furnishing a house you always do it with your current situation in mind. Most people never think when searching for a house that one day you might have to care for a loved one in it. When it comes to looking after a loved one it can be a distressing time so then the last thing you want is the stress of finding a new home that is better suited for your needs or the stress to the loved one you are caring for of taking them out of their usual surroundings.

The word 'normal' will not exist to you any more after caring for a loved one. The first thing you will do is try to make it as easy as possible for you and your loved one to get around the house. This may mean moving beds downstairs if they are no longer able to go up the stairs. It may include making walkways wider and removing any trip or slip hazards. You may need to reposition things around the house out of harm's way and reach or you may need to move things so they are in easy reach, depending on what your loved one needs access to during the day. Life should now be about making the daily life for you and your loved one as easy and simple as possible.

If you have lots of expensive items, furnishings and carpets, you may need to put these out of the way or be prepared for them to get damaged. Sometimes a house can seem like a war zone and you can spend more time fixing things and cleaning things up than you do anything else. It may be worth looking into covers, protectors and the best stuff you can use to clean things with. I know you don't want to have to think about all this stuff but if you are house-proud you are really going to need all this information and build an understanding that it's not your loved one's fault if things do get damaged; they aren't doing it on purpose. Things can be replaced and the items that can't be replaced we can't take with us when we are gone. It is the people that are the most important and their smiles, so never give them reason to be upset or make them feel upset over damage caused because of their illness.

One thing to look at is grants and financial support to get adaptations made to your house. It can be a bit of a minefield trying to work out what you may need in the way of grab rails, doors, mats etc. so get assessed by a professional and see what needs doing. Be prepared for your house to be changed, for holes to be drilled in your walls and for grab rails to be everywhere if that's what is needed. Who cares what your house looks like if it makes caring for a loved one easier?

Decor can be repaired and household items can be replaced. It wouldn't bother me if it affected the value of the house, made it look ugly or if people thought the current living situation was weird. I wouldn't care if I had to sleep in the kitchen to make it all work and I had to break all the house rules. I would adapt anything in the house I had to in order to make it work, no matter how inconvenient that made things for me. I would change and fit my life and routine completely around the one I was caring for, no matter how silly it would make me look. My main aim was to make my mum happy and confident. The last thing I would want to do was embarrass my mum or make it look like she was the odd one out. The changing of the daily routine and the house wasn't just to make her safe but to make her happy and to take as much stress out of any process as humanly possible.

When caring for a loved one you need a daily routine to make sure that you give the best level of care possible and that everything gets done right. However, when you are caring for someone like my mum with dementia you have to be able to adapt quickly as it can be quite an unpredictable illness. So you can go into your day with a plan of what is going to happen and what you are going to do but at any moment you have to be ready to change and adapt and deal with the situation you have on your hands.

I would adapt my daily schedule around my mum so I would find places near to where I needed to take my mum to do things and get things from, even if these weren't my favourite places or the best places. I would try not to fix specific times to be places or see people as the situation with mum could change every hour. By not making plans I never let anyone down and could then just go places and see people when I got the chance. When I had to set times for things I would often find myself having to cancel or change the times or not attend.

I enjoyed playing games with mum to keep her mind active and to give mum some enjoyment and sense of achievement. One of our favourites was Scrabble. To play this, I had to constantly adapt the rules as mum deteriorated but we never stopped playing. We wouldn't keep score and if mum needed a letter to finish a word I would find it for her and give it to her. If mum had a word but it didn't combine with any letters on the board I would let her put it up separate and then join it in to the rest when there was space. When doing activities with your loved one you should always be looking at ways you can adapt it to make it the best, most fun, situation for your loved one. It never mattered that nobody won and the rules kept on changing as mum enjoyed it and could get a sense of achievement from it and that's all I ever wanted.

Mum and I used to like going on walks in the countryside. We would walk for ages over all kinds of terrain. However, as mum's condition deteriorated we weren't able to go on those big hikes that we used to but it didn't stop us going out. Instead, we started sticking to flatter routes and only go part of the distance we used to go. Everything was about making the most stress-free event as possible because if the person you are caring for is less stressed then you in turn will be less stressed and the more the both of you will be able to enjoy it.

When doing things like these it is important not to get downhearted that things are changing or going downhill. I know it's easy for me to say that but I have been exactly where you are now. The difficulty of the challenge achieved isn't what is important; neither is doing exactly the same thing you did yesterday, last week or the year before that. The only thing that needs to remain the same is your and your loved one's smile. Always think about the outcomes and the reason for doing something rather than what you are actually doing.

Don't be afraid to adapt your likes and what you like doing to fit in with caring for your loved one. If you start enjoying the same music, programmes and activities as them you will find everything feels more like having fun and enjoying time with your loved one than feeling like doing something that they would like at the cost of your own wishes. The more you can see them having fun, and the more they can see you having fun, the better the experience will be for both of you.

Life changes but it is important that you never let it change you, your feelings towards the world around you and how you attack life. You can't control what is going to change around you and how it is going to change but you can control how you react to it. Be on your toes, be ready for anything and always try your best to make every day as brilliant and as special as the last. Do this and you can't go far wrong.

CHAPTER SEVENTEEN

Research

Research is an important tool when caring for someone. Never just accept what you are told without questioning it and researching it. The better researched you are the better equipped you are to deal with what is going on. It is important when you go into situations to know as much as you can and be as well-informed as you possibly can be. Without research you can be putting all your heart and soul into caring but you might not be caring in the right ways or doing the right things, which may mean all your hard work is for nothing or you could be making things worse for the one you are caring for.

The two areas you need to spend your time researching are how to care for someone with the specific condition that your loved one has and what is the best thing medically for them (what surgery they should be having, if any; what treatment they should be getting; what medication they should be getting, and so forth). Without research you can't expect to change things or improve things. I would hate to know after my loved one had died that there was something I could have done differently or better to give them a better quality of life. Research is one way you can make sure that doesn't happen to you and that you don't end up with a lot of regrets later in life.

I know that for many people when their loved one passes on they spend a lot of time researching, trying to find someone to blame or trying to improve lives for others still suffering with that condition. Doing that is all well, and good and I know they are coping mechanisms, but I would much rather spend time whilst my loved one was still alive to make things better. Each day, try to carve out time to do some research or ask friends and family members to do some for you on specific areas. I know it is hard to balance doing this with the actual caring side but I think it is so worth it and leads to long-term gain. I know when you are researching you will be thinking to yourself that you should be spending that time caring but the positives of it outweigh the negatives.

When researching you need the gift of discernment and the conviction to keep wading through. When you first start putting a search into Google or visit the library for the first time you will be hit with a ton of information and you won't know where to start. Don't be put off, take a deep breath and go through it systematically. Don't give up because if you give up you may miss out on that important piece of information or advice that you needed. You need to turn yourself into a student of the condition the loved one you are caring for is suffering from and a student of the art of caring.

Try to be level-headed and balanced when researching things. Never dismiss anything you find out of hand but on the other hand don't fully subscribe to a theory without testing it and checking it first. There are going to be lots of areas where there is no right or wrong answer as a lot of it will be opinion-based. I try to take bits and pieces from different sources as I believe lots of people do talk sense but aren't 100% perfect in their views and opinions. When online, don't just listen to experts; also listen to people who are in a similar position to you, see what worked for them and give that a try.

The thing to remember is that you are different from any other carer and the loved one you are caring for is different from anyone else. It's a case of fitting the knowledge and information you find during research into your daily life, not trying to fit your daily life into what you have researched. If you spend hours or days researching and it just leads to you tweaking something small about your daily routine or the way you act then it is time well spent.

Don't be afraid to question what you are reading online. Test it, see if it holds up; see if anyone else online subscribes to the same theory or ideas. An indicator if something works can be if other people are doing the same thing. This isn't a golden, unbreakable rule but something to consider. Take your info to a professional to see what they say and if you truly believe in the info have the conviction to carry it out in your own life, regardless of what others say.

Research shouldn't just be a one-way street – interact with the information you are finding. Contact the person who wrote what you are reading, ask questions, get further advice. Put questions out there online and see if anyone responds. This process is about talking as well as listening. Research and theories can change on a daily basis, so never be afraid of checking the same sites regularly and going back over things you have already read to see if they are still true.

Never think you know everything or know more than others. When caring for someone you can't be proud. If you are doing something wrong or hold beliefs that are wrong you have to be willing to change and adapt. Don't be stubborn and hold on to things just because you think you are right. No matter how long you research you will never know everything, not even close, regardless of how long you research.

Be specific in your research, looking for small points that are important to you. Try not to fill your head with too much irrelevant stuff if you can help it. The more specific your searches on the Internet and in libraries the more likely you are to find relevant stuff that you want or need to read. The more generic your searches are the harder it will be to get the knowledge you are searching for. The more thought you can put in before you search the better and easier your research will be.

A good tip is if you see anything on TV, read anything in a newspaper or hear anything on the radio regarding caring or the condition you are caring for, note it down right away. It is so easy to forget about it or forget some of it; writing it down makes researching it later much easier. When you are caring for a loved one with a specific condition you will tend to hear more stuff about it in the news as your ears naturally prick up when you hear something about it when they didn't before when you weren't going through the situation you are currently going through.

Never be afraid to bring up caring or the condition of the loved one you are caring for in conversation with anyone. Sometimes you can get gems of information from people you would least expect. Lots of people have a lot of life experience to give and may have been through things or worked in professions linked to what you are dealing with but without bringing it up in conversation you will never find that out.

Research is a very up and down process. Some days you could search for hours and get nothing then some days the first thing you look at has a ton of helpful information. Prepare yourself for this, as it can be soul-destroying at times. Just remember that the information is out there waiting for you to discover it but sometimes you need a bit of patience as well. Every time you uncover something that turns out useless it brings you closer to finding something useful. Also, sometimes something that seems like its useless today may come in handy later down the track so no research is ever wasted, even if it doesn't generate what you want it to at the time. Knowledge gained today also helps you better at discerning what is relevant and gives you a wider understanding of information you uncover tomorrow. At times it can seem a bit like a giant jigsaw puzzle you are trying to put together.

Don't go into research with expectations. Try to keep your mind open to everything. Don't set out with an agenda of trying to prove or disprove something. Don't expect to find all the answers you are looking for as many times research will throw up more questions than answers, but that's ok as it encourages you to think more about the subject you are studying. Just remember above all not to lose sight of why you are doing it and what good research could actually help you do. Remember these things and you can't go too far wrong.

CHAPTER EIGHTEEN

Advice

Advice is very easily dispensed at times but sometimes very hard to take on board or to put into action. When you hear advice you can agree with it wholeheartedly and take it all in and in that moment be motivated to put it in to action but as soon as you move away from that conversation or that book it can easily be forgotten. Hearing advice is easy, it is all around us, but actually putting it into practice can be very hard, from the simplest things to the biggest life changes.

If you do have the strength to put advice into action, keeping it up can be the next challenge. Fresh from hearing advice, you can rush home and start implementing it – but as the number of days grows from the day you heard the advice, you can fall back into old ways or stop doing whatever it was you were advised to do. If you don't see instant results you don't get that reward, so you give up and are not patient enough to give it a longer try. If the advice takes a lot of effort on a daily basis you may not have the internal strength to do it every day, especially if it means sacrificing something else to do it. If the advice you have been given asks you to do something that might look strange or is a bit different, you may not have the bravery and confidence to do it on a regular basis; it might just feel a bit too weird and awkward.

You can spend your whole life listening to advice and not act on a single bit, which would be a life wasted. I'm not saying act on every bit of advice you are ever given but eventually you have to choose some advice to follow or to give a go or else you might as well not bother listening to any advice.

Not acting on advice can be a pride thing: it is natural to think you know best and to be self-sufficient and not want help from anyone. We are all raised a certain way, which forms the way we deal with the world, and these ways are very hard to break as they are so ingrained into our being. Sometimes in life we just don't want to hear advice so we don't listen or we start having a go at the people giving the advice as we think they don't know what we are going through. The phrase that comes up often is that "you're a fine one to talk" or "you don't know what it's like for us." I think both of these are excuses because the right advice is the right advice no matter who it comes from. When listening to things it should be about listening to and judging the advice given, not where it is coming from.

Picking the right advice to follow is tricky and what might be right for you might not be the same for somebody else. There may be lots of advice that is right for you and you may need to follow it all. However, some advice may not work with other bits you are given, so you may need to not implement some right and good advice at times as it doesn't quite work or fit with the rest of the advice you are trying to follow.

One thing that is important is to clarify all advice that you want to use to make sure you understand it right so that you can follow it right. There is nothing worse than getting the wrong end of the stick or not understanding something properly. Once you find advice that you like, ask questions of it, and if it is something somebody has told you, write it down. When somebody says something it is very easy to misremember it and think they said something different. It is just that subtle difference in what they said and what you heard that could change advice completely, so be careful with this.

Advice is all about timing: receiving it at the right time to hear it and hearing it at the right time to implement it. We go through times in our life when we don't want to hear certain things and are closed off to it or we don't have the strength to hear it. We also go through times when we get advice when it is too late to help our situation, either because we waited too long to get advice or we just didn't hear it in time. The right advice at the right time in the right place can literally change your life or the lives of those around you.

The key thing is, don't waste or miss out on good advice. Some advice you get lucky enough to hear more than once in your lifetime but with a lot you may hear it only once, and after it is forgotten about, it can never help you again. I would rather be the person that listened then tried and failed rather than the one that never listened and never tried and never had any hope of changing or improving their situation.

If you ever get good advice that works, pass it on; don't keep it to yourself. By passing it on you can help many people for years to come. The chances are that the person you heard it from was just doing the same thing: they heard it somewhere and if they hadn't passed it on you wouldn't have heard about it and it wouldn't have helped you. Passing on advice is easy: it doesn't take long, doesn't take much effort, and if you share it with a friend the reason they may listen to it and implement it is because it came from you. If they had heard it from someone else they might not have bothered.

Giving your own advice to others takes confidence. Many people are scared to do so in case it is wrong, as they don't want to seem stupid or advise someone to do something for them to go and do it and for it to not work. Some people are over-confident when they give advice, reporting their advice more as fact than an opinion when advice can at times have no bearing on fact. When giving your own advice you should preface it by saying this is your advice and you are free to take it if you wish. Doing this means that the person knows that it is coming from you based on your experience and if it doesn't work for the person you are giving the advice to you haven't given it over as fact. It is the listener's responsibility what they do with it, not yours. So if they do it wrong or don't get results it is not your fault.

I think you need to be brave and share as much as you can with others whenever you can. It may be just one phrase or sentence you say that unlocks some new information or advice for someone else. They may not take on board everything you say but your way of saying it or the wording you use can spark something in the person you are talking to. It may be that the person takes your advice in a way you didn't think of and gets great results or benefits from it. When giving advice you will sometimes be surprised by the results. Experience is the greatest builder for advice, so go out and experience as much as you can. There is something you can learn from every experience and a piece of advice can be formed from it.

Gaining advice is like benefiting from someone else's tries and failures as well as other people's experiences. You will never have time in life to experience everything so listening to people who have experienced things that you haven't can be the greatest way to learn. If you can't afford or don't have the time to try and fail at things, talk to someone who has. If you do have time to try and fail at things, never be afraid to fail. It may be that your failure changes the world and teaches you more than any success. Your failure may also stop many more people failing in the future. However, if you are going to fail, try to fail at something that someone hasn't failed at before or fail in a way that no one else has before. When giving advice, if you can make it relevant to real life and speak from experience and share your experience then people are more likely to pay attention and remember it. The way you give advice is key to whether someone will listen to it, remember it and put it in to action.

CHAPTER NINETEEN

Support

Never be afraid to ask for support or to go and seek it out. If someone offers you support, take it. Don't feel like you have to say 'no' or be too proud to accept help. If other people offer support, you are entitled to take them up on their offer. When the chips are down you will be surprised how far people will go to support you. Don't forget, there are people in this world who like supporting other people and are really good at it, so don't be afraid to let them. Don't think about burdening others because sometimes what you think is a burden to someone another person wouldn't see as a burden at all. Remember not to apply your own thoughts on what are burdens and support to other people.

If someone says they can't support you there will always be another one that will. Sometimes it is good to find out who will support you and who won't so you know in which areas and people in your life it is worth investing energy. Remember, you don't want just anyone supporting you: you want people who truly care about you and your loved one, people who are reliable and people you can trust. It may take you a while to find out who these people are and it may not be clear for some time but when you do it is a valuable feeling to know who these treasured people are. With people that provide you with day-to-day support, you need reliable people.

Support can come in all different forms from all different kinds of people and places, so you need to be open to it at all times and ready to receive it. Something you might not see as support now may turn out when you look back on life to being the most supportive thing that ever happened to you. Getting support with the little things in life is what can make the big difference. Whether you like it or not, whether you know about it or not, there are people out there who are supporting you and people who want to support you.

There is no weakness in asking for support. If you feel that is shows weakness then you aren't thinking things through logically and I think that is a real weakness. Asking for support is not a slight or negative comment on what you have been doing and does not reflect badly on your efforts. It only shows that you want the best for the person you are caring for and yourself. It shows you are wise enough to realise in what areas of your caring life you aren't the best and need support. No carer is brilliant at everything; every carer needs support in at least one area, sometimes many.

This might sound crazy but sometimes when you are caring for someone it is a nice feeling to be able to offer someone else some support. It can make you feel valued and that you are making a difference to others. When you are the one being supported a lot it can be quite therapeutic to support someone else for a moment as a break from what you are going through. This is why I like things like carers groups as it can be a great feeling to support others and it can really build togetherness between you and other carers, whilst making you feel less alone, less scared and less isolated. Supporting someone else can also give you more confidence to do more in your own caring situation. Supporting others can also help put your life into perspective a bit, to see you aren't the only one going through what you are going through and no matter what you are going through there is always someone better off and someone worse off. I know it's hard to see it at times but it is important to realise it.

Don't put off getting support. Don't struggle from one day to the next wishing you had support. The quicker you get support the easier it becomes to accept it and for it to make a big impact in your life and the life of the person you are caring for. If you let yourself get too stressed or let the health of the person you are caring for deteriorate it can be hard for the support to make as big a difference as it would have earlier. The longer you put off asking for support the harder it becomes to ask. You think to yourself that you have survived this long doing what you are doing so what harm is there in struggling on for another day or do I really need support?

No one will ever laugh at you for asking for support. Never see what you are going through as trivial. People will understand and want to help you. Nothing is more comforting than being helped by someone, so never be afraid to get that experience. Get yourself that releasing feeling of asking for help and receiving it; it is so liberating. It feels great once you have asked for support. You feel stronger after you have done it and proud that you had the courage to ask for it. Everyone has the ability to help someone in some way. It is going to be different for different people but it is something we all have inside us.

Sometimes you may be a bit overwhelmed by the level of support that comes in and the number of people wanting to support you. It can sometimes feel like you are losing control and can be scary at times. Just remember that you can structure the way you get support and the way they support you. You need to schedule the support in a way that is best for the one you are caring for. Work out who the right people are to give you support and which areas they should give you support in. You may not want too many different people around or in the house, so try to devise a way that works for you.

The one time you do need to be careful when accepting support is when someone wants to help in an area they aren't experienced in or don't know anything about. People will think they can do things or that things are easy when it actually turns out that they can't do it. Don't be afraid to ask questions of those offering support or to teach them how to do something if it is something you know how to do. Support doesn't always mean getting in someone better than you in a certain area; it can just be about getting someone in to do something to free up your time for someone else. Find what these things are and teach them to others whenever you get a chance. When someone is new to the house, spend a while getting them acclimatized. Show them around, show them where things are and then watch them carry out their support tasks. This will give you peace of mind when you leave them to get on with things by themselves and will make sure that the helper is giving the best and right support. When support first comes in you are going to have to invest some time in the short term, so life may get a bit busier or harder for a little while, but the long-term gain outweighs the short term pain.

Whatever you end up doing, always remember to thank people if they give or offer support, even if you don't accept it. For some people it's a big step to offer support so never look at it lightly. Never expect support but always appreciate it. When someone helps another human being it should be applauded. You can't always change the world but if you can change the world for one person then you have done something amazing and something you should be proud of forever.

Through asking for support you can make friends that last a lifetime. One of the things about caring is the isolation it can cause so this is one good way of counteracting this. Having someone else in the house can help you mentally as you see someone from the outside world on a regular basis who you can talk to and with. By having people in your house it also means that there is a regular check on you and your loved one so you won't go days and days without help or support, which I think improves the safety of you and your loved one. That can only be a positive thing. There are so many ways that getting support can help, most of which you may never realise.

CHAPTER TWENTY

Giving Back

My mum and I had a very special relationship. We knew each other's dreams, shared the same likes in music, TV and hobbies and would do anything to help each other. A lot of the things I still like today I like because my mum liked them and I just copied her. The football team I support and the music I listen to are all because she liked them first. If it wasn't for mum I don't think I would have been half as interested in football as I am or have achieved the level of success I have in the sport. This is just one of many examples of how mum made me who I am today.

When I was growing up mum would do everything and anything for me. She would walk me to the local primary school and pick me up each day. She would come to all of my sports days and nativity plays and she would help out wherever she could in school, from helping take our school swimming at the local pool to coming along as a helper on school field trips. Mum tried to be as active and as helpful as she could in my schooling. When I moved up to secondary there were two stops for the school bus in our village and they wanted to send me to the nearest one. But mum argued and got them to let me on the bus a little further walk away because it was seen as a cooler bus stop and I wanted to get on that one. On days I didn't want to catch the bus mum would drive me the three miles to school and pick me up at home time. She never made me go to school if I didn't want to and was always on hand to help out with any homework. Mum even did some of the homework for me to make my life easier. I remember in textiles we had to make a bag so mum did the sewing for me because I couldn't do it. That was the kind of mum she was.

As a young boy I was a member of the cubs and there was a *writing of English* badge that I wanted. I had to do a piece of writing and because I wasn't any good at it she did it for me and I got the badge. I loved collecting the badges in cubs and had an armful of them on my Cubs uniform. Mum knew how much I wanted every badge so to the rescue she came.

Living in a small village three miles away from the school meant I couldn't just walk and see friends, so whenever I wanted to see someone or go to something mum would drop what she was doing and take me. To get a bit of money when I was younger I got myself a paper round but instead of me doing it by foot or by bike, mum would drive me around to make it easier on me. Everyone else that did it didn't have their parents doing it but on a cold day and with a heavy bag it was awesome to be driven around. When there was something I wanted to do mum would always drive. When I wanted to become a football referee mum would drive me every Monday for 10 weeks down to a town 12 miles away for me to do the course. From then on she would drive me around Cornwall and Devon every Saturday for football. For my work experience at school I wanted to work at Devon County Football Association so for five days in a row mum would drive me to Newton Abbot, which was a 100 mile round trip, and she would do that every morning to drop me off and every afternoon to pick me up.

During the summer holidays mum would take me up every day to summer training camps at the nearest professional football club, which was Plymouth Argyle about 25 miles away. She would drop me off in the morning go back home then come and pick me up again in the evening, which probably completely messed her day around but she didn't care.

Mum would always be encouraging me or telling me about ~opportunities she had found for me. Mum would always take an interest in what I was watching or what I was doing. There were not many hours outside of school that we weren't doing something together – even walking the dog, doing the dishes or doing the shopping.

When I left University and went into the workplace I would ring mum every lunchtime to see how she was and sometimes I would ring two or three times a day, especially when I knew she was at home by herself. I would always make sure on the phone that I was as positive as possible and spent every call trying to make her smile and to feel good about herself. I would start every call by saying, "How is my favourite mum in the entire world?" and would end it by saying "see you in a while, crocodile" as she loved animals. I will never forget those calls.

Whenever I was out and about I would always be looking for presents for mum or small things I could buy her, from her favourite chocolate to a CD or a book she might like. I would spend my last penny on mum, always felt great giving her something and seeing her smile and brightening up her day. As the illness developed I would always be thinking of things that would be practical for her or things that would stimulate her mind; just anything to make her day the best it could possibly be.

Even when I was an adult living at home mum would always make sure she was up before I got up to make me breakfast and to make me lunch. I didn't ask – she just did it because she wanted to be the best mum. She waved me off to work every day and when I got home she would cook dinner, do the dishes and wash any clothes I needed washing. There wasn't an area of life where she didn't help me.

I think mum did this because subconsciously she thought "there might come a time when I need someone to look after me" or she did it because she thought she might die young so wanted to spend as much time with me as she could and have as strong a relationship as possible. I will never know the real reasons but all I know is that she made an amazing mum and was so awesome in her role as a mother. Mum didn't need to do anything for me because I was always going to care for her, no matter what, if the situation arose, which sadly it did. I wanted to spend my life being my mum's best friend but in the end it turned into best friend and carer. Although I wish more than anything that this never happened and mum was still with us all fit and healthy, I am glad that I got the chance in a very small way to give back what she gave to me by helping to care for her and making her life as fun and bearable as possible.

Before the illness I just thought giving back would be coming down to see mum from time to time and ringing her up every day on the phone. I never thought it would be giving back as I did. That's the thing with life; you never know how or when you will be able to or have to give something back. But I always knew I was going to try to be as good to mum as she was to me because this was the least I could do in return for everything she did for me.

CHAPTER TWENTY-ONE

Making the Best of Things

When something so bad happens – like my mum's illness – it can take every ounce of happiness from you and bring such sadness. But no matter how bad things get I always feel the most important thing is to make the best of it. Even though mum's condition was progressive and we knew where it was going to end up, we tried to make the best of every day we had and make things the best for mum that we could. We couldn't show mum sadness; we wanted her days to be happy days, so I would save my tears for my bedroom and tried to make any situation with mum funny and happy and made sure I was always smiling in her presence.

Mum's condition meant there were many limitations on what she could do. I would work round what mum couldn't do and focus on what she could do and we'd do that. We would take the simplest things and make them as fun as possible, from throwing a ball to moving around the house. We would make a game out of anything. Any time mum achieved something we would praise her and would celebrate even the smallest of successes. Some were things that most people do without thinking but to mum they were huge and took a lot of concentration to do.

As soon as we got the diagnosis we booked a family holiday to Australia, a country we had never been to but one mum always wanted to visit as it played host to many of her favourite things. Whatever it cost, it didn't matter. We just wanted mum to do everything in life she wanted to do. I took three weeks off work and mum, dad and I went to Australia, cramming as much into three weeks as we could. Mum loved the *Crocodile Hunter* TV series with Steve Irwin so we had to go to his Australia Zoo where it was filmed We spent two days there, making sure we saw every last bit of it. Mum also loved the TV show *Neighbours* so we went to some of the areas it was filmed. Finally, one of the places she had always wanted to visit was Uluru – or Ayres Rock, as some people call it – so we got an internal flight over there as well, making sure mum got to do everything she wanted to do.

We took mum to Emirates Stadium to see Arsenal, a team she had supported from a young age and got me supporting. We had been to their old Highbury stadium when mum was well but hadn't been to the new stadium together. We took mum to see friends and family in different places in the UK, to the theatre and to concerts, including one of her favourites, Glen Campbell.

We wanted to make sure mum had the chance to do everything she wanted to do. We didn't want her condition to stop her from being able to experience these things. I thought that all the new experiences and places would help stimulate her brain and – although she couldn't enjoy these things to the maximum as others might – that she would remember some bits and enjoy some bits of the experiences. Whenever we went anywhere new I would always research and plan the trip ahead to make it the best possible experience, whether it was a big or small place we were going to.

It was quite easy for me to make the most of things with mum, as I never accepted during her conditions that she might go into care or die from illnesses related to dementia, although I did make sure I enjoyed every day I had with mum. Mum was still just mum to me and she and I would enjoy anything as long as we were in each other's company. No matter how bad things got I didn't panic, I just kept going and focused on being positive, which was my coping mechanism.

I tried to pack as much as I could into every day with mum. Although I didn't get as much time as I would like with mum due to all my other commitments, this made me more determined to make the best of the time I had. I did not want to dwell on what was happening and give my-self time to think and get depressed so I was always doing things when I was with mum. Then when I wasn't with mum I was thinking of things I could do with her or ways I could do things differently.

I would always put a positive spin on everything instead of thinking about the negative things to do with mum's illness. If it were not for mum's illness I would have probably left home after university and not come back to live but because of mum's condition I stayed. That meant I got the chance to spend a lot of time with her, something that most people miss out on, and I had a bond with my mum that very few have with their mums, which were two major positives for me. I actually got the chance to give back and to try in some small way to repay what my mum had done for me since I was born. I would rather be living at home and having an amazing relationship with my mum than living elsewhere and having a bad relationship with my parents.

I enjoyed helping mum and took a great pride in it. I wanted to be the best I could be for my mum as she deserved it and needed me to be it. In the early stages I would love taking mum out in the car or for a coffee locally. These trips got less and less as it progressed but because we had made the most in this area during the early stages we could look back on these moments with fond memories.

Whenever I was out and about and bumped into people I would always say things were good or not as bad as they actually were. I didn't want people worrying because I knew the pain I felt inside and I didn't want anyone else to feel that same pain. Your close friends and family want to hear how you are doing but people in the street and casual acquaintances don't want to know your real life story. When I was out of the house I wanted to be distracted and I didn't want to go back through what was happening at home and not talking about it was my way of making the best of the time I had outside the house.

I would always make sure I made the best of the time when I was away from the house. I would organise my commitments so I could get the most done in the shortest space of time possible. I would be efficient and make meetings as quick as they could be. I would pack up early when coaching and try to make sure I got away from sessions early or on time. I would always try to bunch appointments geographically so I could go from one to the other quickly. Everything I could do at home I did to try to avoid trips away from mum but what wasn't avoidable I would make as quick as possible, and if I could get out of something and not attend it I would. I would also use technology where I could, doing meetings over conference calls, emails, Skype etc. so I could contribute whilst not having to leave mum and be able to look after mum at the same time. I can remember many an evening sitting with mum on the sofa, laptop on my lap, phone in my ear and proving that men *can* actually multi-task.

I think when life is bad the ability to make the best of things is very important. I think it helps you to care better for the person you are caring for and it stops you wallowing in the sadness or pain of the situation you are in. You have lots of time later to do that but during a situation like I had with mum every minute was vitally important and I am so happy that I handled it in the way I did.

Making the best of everything is about appreciating just the smallest of things and looking for that positive to take from a situation. Sometimes you have to search really hard but those small positives or those wonderful moments are what make the long periods of pain bearable. Without these things I don't know if I would have had the strength to carry on and get out of bed every morning. Remember to concentrate on what you can do and not what you can't do – and the same for the person you are caring for; concentrate on what they can do, not what they can't do. What they can do may get less each day but just appreciate what you have whilst you have it.

CHAPTER TWENTY-TWO

A Calling

For many years I didn't know what I was put on this earth to do or what to do with my life. I have always believed that I was put on the earth for a special reason but I have not known what that reason was for so long. When mum got diagnosed with dementia I didn't even think, I didn't even stop, I just went into caring mode – and without a second thought I knew I was going to dedicate my life to looking after my mum. It was so natural, so right and so instinctive that I truly believe that is what I was put on earth to do.

When people think they were put on earth to do great things they probably think that will be making money, being famous, doing something creative or doing something that changes the world. After what happened with my mum, I now see great things don't mean any of that. Doing great things is about changing the world for one person, about caring for others, about showing love to others. To do great things you don't need qualifications, training or money, just an internal strength. The greatest things can be achieved with your character, personality, strength and mind. Some people spend life listening to their internal thoughts and feelings and act upon them when the time comes. Sadly, so many people try to run away from their thoughts and feelings, and when tough times come or hard decisions need to be made they shy away or ignore instincts.

Some people go out there and find their calling; some people just wait until the situation comes to them, knowing that one day it will happen. Before my mum's illness I had tried in so many ways to achieve in various areas but with limited success. I would get part of the way there but never get to where I wanted to go. In my younger days I would set very high standards or ideals on what success was; the goals in some cases were quite unobtainable. Sometimes I think you try to force things too much when you aren't sure what your calling is. I think everyone wants a calling and that everyone wants to know what that calling is. Sometimes, if you try to force it like I did, you can spend years wasting times pursuing success for no reason or long-term gain. I think it is better to search from within first before you spend precious time going down the wrong path.

When you do find your calling it just feels right. Nothing made me prouder in life than caring for my mum. I felt so important and like I was making a real difference in the world, feelings I have never had whilst doing anything else. Your calling isn't about money, fame or success, it is about the feeling you get whilst you are doing it.

Your calling may not be easy, your calling may not be rewarding, it may not bring happiness, it may not change the world but you know it will all be worth it and it gives you purpose and that feeling of success that only comes with knowing that you are doing what you are put on earth to do.

CHAPTER TWENTY-THREE

A Mission

When caring for someone in your family you can see it as your mission to improve their life and to look after them. It can feel at times that you are going into battle for them and that it is you against the world. You feel you are going to change everything and you aren't going to stop until your mission is complete. You know what your goal is and you go about every day doing things and finding out things to help you achieve your goal.

When on a mission you will stop at nothing to achieve it, you will be focused and dedicated to achieve it. On a mission you might recruit others to help you and have the biggest army or you might not trust anyone else to have the same passion and work rate, so you may want to go it alone.

Missions are normally born out of injustice or a feeling of being wronged. This is very similar to when caring for someone, as you start thinking that your loved one shouldn't have to suffer the injustice of what they are suffering. This could mean that if you don't think a doctor is helping, you may try to find another doctor or get a 'better' doctor and stop at nothing to get a doctor that you like for your loved one. If there isn't enough funding for support, you may go round asking for funding for specialist treatment, writing and emailing and phoning everyone you can think of. If the government aren't doing enough to support it or support the illness your loved one is suffering with in the right way, you may take to political campaigning.

To get support for your mission you may need some publicity, so that might mean engaging with the local and national press. Starting up and writing for websites and social media may be more the answer in the technological world we live in. Publicity may mean going out and talking to people face to face about it and arranging events to draw attention to your cause. When caring for your loved one it may give you the passion to make a difference, not just for your loved one but for other people suffering with the same thing – and if it were not for your loved one suffering with a specific illness you wouldn't have known anything about it or be passionate about it. You then try to get other people who aren't affected by something to feel passionately about that cause but this can be easier said than done at times. It can feel quite frustrating when you meet someone and they don't know anything something and don't seem to care about it, even though it is so devastating to you and affects every bit of your life.

CHAPTER TWENTY-FOUR

A Reason for Living

When mum got diagnosed with dementia she became my reason for living. My life was no longer about me or living for myself, it was all for my mum. Mum was my world and my everything for all my years growing up but now not only was she this she was now someone to whom I could dedicate my life. Everything else became a distant second priority or not a priority at all.

For many people, when something like this happens it becomes a reason to cry and a reason for sadness and, for a few, a reason not to live any more and to take their own life. When bad things start happening you can't blame people for feeling down or depressed but if you want to help you can't stay that way for long. Some people say that when someone starts caring for someone and stops doing anything else that they aren't living any more. I personally think that's a load of rubbish. I think that when you care for a loved one you are living for someone else and living with more purpose than you did before it happened.

It's quite interesting after you have cared for a loved one to look back and think what your reasons were for living before you started caring for them. You will either not be able to think of any or, if you do think of any, they will seem so trivial and rubbish. I think whether you are caring for someone or not you need to have a clear reason for living and

105

remind yourself of it every day. Reasons for living can be for other people, to achieve goals or just to feel a certain way or do a certain thing. Something that may seem trivial to you as a reason to live might be huge to another person so never mock anyone else for their reason for living.

It's when you don't have a reason to live or can't find one that life gets hard. This is when people become depressed, stop doing things and stop finding reasons to go out of the house. This can lead to a whole host of issues and, if extreme enough, can lead to people taking their own lives. I think people need to have a feeling that they have something to do, that they can do and that there are things out there for them to enjoy. I think that without this reason for living to hang on to it can be very bad and affect your thought patterns and your emotions.

The one thing you have to be sure to do is to not hold on to this reason for living when life changes. If your reason for living is wrapped up in someone else, if they move out of your life you have to be ready and willing to find a new reason for living. If you don't do this then life afterwards can be very hard and without that reason to live it can set you in a negative tailspin.

CHAPTER TWENTY-FIVE

Keep Smiling

One thing you can never afford to lose is your smile. Life can be pretty uncontrollable at times and many bad things can happen that you can't stop but if you can approach it all with a smile on your face it will give you the strength to keep on fighting and putting one foot in front of the other. A smile is such a precious gift but it can so easily be lost.

A smile is one of the best things in the world to share. You will be surprised how often when you smile that people around you start smiling. One person can start the most amazing smile wave that sends a bit of happiness and positivity into the lives of so many. The only thing you need to do to share a smile is smile yourself; you don't have to give it away and you don't lose anything by doing it.

Never let anyone else stop you from smiling or make you think you can't or shouldn't or have no reason to smile. There is always a reason to smile. I found that when I smiled I thought better about myself, the world around me and what was happening. The act of smiling just made me feel happy inside. A smile won't solve the world's problems but it will make solving them in a rational manner a lot easier.

Never feel bad about smiling. Smiling doesn't mean that you don't feel bad about the situation. You can smile and still care about a situation. You can be sympathetic, empathetic and compassionate and still smile. On the flipside, don't make yourself feel bad if you aren't feeling bad. Emotions will come and go. You don't have to make yourself feel a certain way; life will do that to you.

The worst thing you can do is feel bad about not being sad. Just because life is bad it doesn't mean that you should stop finding joy and happiness in different things. I think it's even more important to find reasons to smile when things are going badly. If you don't want other people to feel sorry for you, you have to keep smiling.

When life is crashing down around you being able to smile and face everything positively can help you cope and deal with everything in an efficient manner. Sometimes, when we get upset and stressed, it can lead to wrong decisions or decisions prompted by strong emotions. It can lead to you losing your rag, taking out your temper on people around you and becoming quite unhappy yourself. Stress and unhappiness can lead to you not knowing what decision to make when you are faced with a stressful situation or could lead you to not taking any decision at all and fleeing from the responsibility.

In sad times you can find yourself smiling at the most random things and sometimes for no reason. Sometimes you can smile at the most inappropriate of times because of everything that is going on but don't feel embarrassed about it or ashamed of it. Sometimes you can find things darkly comical. Its not being disrespectful to people, it is just another coping mechanism that you should not be ashamed of.

Never be annoyed when other people in your family or friendship groups are smiling during bad times in your family. It is OK for them to smile, never tell them that they should or shouldn't be smiling; let them handle the situation in their own way. Just because their way of handling things is different from yours doesn't make it wrong.

One thing to remember is that if you asked the person you were caring for they wouldn't want you to be upset, they would want you to be happy. If the person you were caring for knew you were unhappy it would probably make them more unhappy and they have enough to deal with. Keeping on smiling shows them that you are handling the situation and making the best of life. The person you are caring for probably already thinks you give up way too much for them but if they knew caring was making you unhappy as well it would hurt them so much. Everything you do should be to provide the best care and environment for your loved one and smiling should be part of that plan.

If you want to support others in your family through the process of caring for a loved one you have no choice but to keep on smiling. If they see you being unhappy it will mean they try to look after and support you, not the other way round. There is great strength in smiling and smiling in bad situations means you are made of tough stuff.

Smiling isn't about thinking life is great or being happy with the situation you face. Smiling isn't showing that you think what is happening to your loved one is trivial or nothing to worry about. Smiling is about making every day count and making every day the best and happiest day it can be in the situation you find yourself in. Situations change, sometimes on a daily or hourly basis. You can't control the world around you but you can control how you react to it. You have the power to make today a better day. You don't need any training or qualifications, it's just something we are born with the ability to do – and that's smile.

CHAPTER TWENTY-SIX

Attitudes

One thing that I hope will change in the future is the attitude towards people suffering from mental illnesses. If you are suffering from mental health issues it seems there is less compassion out there from the general public than if you were going through something physical that people can see. When someone is not acting in a way you would expect some people think its OK to call them names or make fun of them instead of thinking they are ill. A lot of people suffering from mental health issues couldn't communicate to the public in a way to let them know they were ill, so they couldn't tell people even if they wanted to, which I am sure most don't.

For those suffering with mental health issues who are still aware of the world around them, calling them names or laughing at them or treating them differently could have a majorly-negative effect on their well-being and their condition. People suffering from mental ill health shouldn't be frightened or embarrassed to try to live as close to 'normal' life as they possibly can. One thing I can't stand is the names and words people use in day-to-day conversation to describe someone who is suffering with mental illness. I hate the terms mental, loopy, funny farm, not all there, not playing with a full deck of cards – and the list goes on and on. Why can't we just say unwell or ill? We do for every other illness.

Our mental health is so fragile we should never underestimate the power of our words and actions towards the subject and people suffering mental illness.

I hate how people suffering with mental illness are seen as people to be frightened of, to move away from and to ignore. Many people suffering with dementia currently were just like you or me for large portions of their life. The only thing that has happened is that they got ill. If you act this way towards people with mental illnesses then other people around you will. It builds this fear and ostracises them even more when they can least afford it and could really do with friends and social interaction.

Something people don't seem to have is patience. Everyone is always rushing to get somewhere or to do something. Not many people these days would be willing to wait patiently in a queue behind someone with mental health issues, who may take longer to do things like buying something from a shop. No one seems to have the time to stop and interact and talk with them. Someone with a mental illness will have enough anxiety or fear going about their day-to-day life so the public shouldn't make it even worse. People need to recognise that any one of us can have to deal with a mental health issue and there is nothing anyone can do about it.

When you see someone in the street suffering with mental health issues put yourself in their shoes for a minute. Whilst you are in a rush to see a friend or to go to work they are just trying to make the best of their day and survive another day. Be careful of the words you speak to people with mental health issues and with friends and colleagues when you talk about mental health. Each and every one of us can play a role in making this world a better place for people with mental health issues.

Holding a conversation with someone suffering from mental health issues can be a challenge and I am not saying it is an easy thing to do but it doesn't mean you shouldn't do it. Just be patient and let them talk as much as possible. Try to go along with what they are saying and listen to them. Forget about what is actually going on in the world and just focus on them. What they are saying may not make sense but they may be enjoying talking to you so it doesn't need to make sense. Remember as well to always be calm and take your time when speaking, as that will help the conversation a lot.

As the level of medical understanding on mental health goes up our consideration as the general public needs to go up. More and more people are affected by mental ill health each day and many studies say that it is on the rise, so the chances are that sometime in your lifetime you, your family or your friends will be affected by it. People with mental health issues don't want to scare you and aren't trying to; it's just that they have a little or no control of their actions or their words any more.

No one asks for or wants to have mental health issues. Although some people's lifestyles have contributed to their current mental health state many had no control over it and have done nothing themselves to cause it. Some mental health issues are genetic, some are pre-determined but many are unavoidable and the people carrying them can go many years without realising they have them.

Some people have mental health issues due to bad things that have happened to them or events they have witnessed in their lives. They might have been abused from a young age; they might have been caught up in a life of drugs and crime. They might just have been in the wrong place at the wrong time to witness something horrific. They might have been mistreated or suffered what they believe to be too much injustice or they might blame themselves for stuff that has happened, like their parents splitting up or for a number of things that happened in their youth.

Or quite simply some people might not have been blessed with the ability to cope with the world around them. This is something many of us take for granted and do without thinking, but for many it is a skill that they lack and it affects so much of their daily life and can lead to a number of mental health issues. So when talking with or interacting with someone with mental health issues, don't blame them, blame the illness!

Another attitude that needs to change is people's attitude to carers and caring. To some, caring for a loved one is seen as a way of escaping life and not having to work or a way of collecting more benefits. Some people take pity on carers and some people don't see caring for someone as being as important as paid jobs the carer could otherwise be doing. Being a carer is the hardest job you could ever have but it is so worthwhile, so rewarding and so life-changing. To me, there aren't many jobs out there that make a difference like caring for another person.

A carer has to give up so much and sacrifice a lot of their own personal dreams and ambitions. People who care for loved ones save this country so much money and they should be commended for it. I think that in many cases the best level of care can be given by loved ones of the person suffering, so where appropriate it should be encouraged – although people shouldn't feel forced into it and it is not their duty or responsibility to be a carer. Don't look down your nose at someone who cares for a loved one; these people are some of the brightest and nicest people I know.

When you see someone out in the street or in a shop caring for someone, try your best to help them and make things as easy for them as possible. The carer's sole focus is the one they are caring for and they may not be quite as focused as you on what is going on around them. The one they are caring for may have a lot of needs and may struggle in social and public settings, so anything you can do will be a huge help. Try not to distract them from what they are doing. If you have spotted something they haven't, tell them right away but when dealing with a situation with their loved one let them do it because they will know best and if they need help they will ask. What you see as helping may be a hindrance, as any change in routine or anything done wrong could make the situation for the carer and their loved one a million times worse.

Don't judge a way a carer cares. What they do may seem strange to you but the thing you need to realise is that every person needs to be cared for slightly differently. That carer has had to adapt what they do in order to get things done and to keep the person they are caring for happy and safe. If you think someone is in danger or being abused then, yes, you need to say something but if you don't see that happening then try to work out why they are doing the things they are doing.

Don't feel embarrassed by carers or the people they are caring for or feel embarrassed on their behalf. Just because something might seem funny, different or not the right way to behave, you don't need to get embarrassed. The carer will already know this and not want you reminding them, and the person they are caring for probably doesn't know or care and wouldn't know how to act in the correct manner in a certain situation.

If you experience mental ill health yourself, don't feel like you're weak and don't be too proud to ask for help if you can. The more we can do to remove the stigma around mental ill health the better. I think we are still in the dark ages on this front and it is one way in which we can make this world better.

CHAPTER TWENTY-SEVEN

Take Nothing for Granted

If there is one thing that caring for my mum taught me it is to take nothing for granted. When you care for someone with dementia it gives you a real appreciation of how easy we have things. Fully fit and healthy people do so many things in a day without even thinking about it, such as feeding, changing and washing ourselves. You never think that one day you won't be able to do these things by yourself and you don't think about how embarrassing it would be if you needed help to do them.

Imagine being totally dependent on someone else for everything. Imagine not being able to or being allowed to do whatever you wanted whenever you wanted. Imagine not being able to remember how to do things or not knowing what is happening in the world around you. Imagine being scared and not knowing what to do or not being able to change it. The quality of life is a very relevant thing and what you quantify as a high quality of life can be different from someone else. To some your life may be brilliant; to some it may be awful.

There are some things in life that you can control and you can choose but dementia is something you can get without causing it by your own actions. I think we all need to enjoy our abilities every day because we never know when they will be taken away from us. Don't look at doing things as a chore when other people who can't do them would love a life of just being able to care for themselves.

Caring for my mum, seeing her getting enjoyment out of the smallest things in life, gave me a real appreciation for what we take for granted. From a game of Scrabble to a game of throw and catch, things we did on a regular basis and things that most people would have got bored with after playing a few times a week, would always make mum smile. She would enjoy these things every day and they would be the highlight of the day.

Regardless of what stage of life and health you are at, just try to make the best out of what you have and what you can do every day. This may change every day but you just have to go with it. You may be able to get back what is lost – and if you can you should invest time in it – but if you can't get back what is lost then don't waste time lamenting it. The key to life is trying to make it the best you can for yourself and for those around you.

There are few constants in this world: health, money, relationships can all change, as will the world around you every day. Sometimes things change for the better, sometimes things change for the worse and sometimes very little changes. Control in life can be an illusion at times and life can seem out of control, so you have to be ready for any- and everything in life and be on your toes always.

Just because you think something is going to happen, it may not; just because you think something you do may cause something, it may not. No one can predict the future and there is very little that is guaranteed to happen in your future. Today is a gift, so enjoy it and do the best you can with it, as no one ever knows what tomorrow will bring. You can think about and plan for the future and affect it but never think something is going to happen. The best thing to do is to hope for things and be appreciative when they do happen.

CHAPTER TWENTY-EIGHT

Be Proactive

Don't wait for situations to happen and think about reacting to them. Try to anticipate and participate. There will be lots of things going on that are out of your control when caring for a loved one but it doesn't mean you have to let life happen to you. The more proactive you are, the better carer you will be and the better level of care you will be able to provide.

If you wait for things to happen it may be too late to do anything to help. It is always easier to try to stop something from happening than trying to fix afterwards. The longer you stay reacting, the bigger the chance of things going wrong or continuing to get worse. I look back at my time caring for mum and there are moments where I wish I had acted faster than I did, as I can see ways in which things could have been different but it is only in hindsight that I have been able to see it.

Being proactive is hard as it forces you out of your comfort zone and forces you to take control, but it is better to go through this than a later life of pain and regrets for not doing anything whilst sitting idly by watching bad things happen. Don't expect others to do everything for you and don't wait for them; stand up yourself and do something.

The earlier you can become proactive the better. The moment you notice something isn't quite right is the moment you need to step in.

Every second, minute, hour and day is precious and can make a huge amount of difference in the life of the person you are caring for, so don't be scared to do something early. Its better to overreact or make a fool of yourself if you think something is wrong rather than waiting to find out something is actually wrong and you could have done something to help.

Being proactive can mean many things. It can mean arming yourself with as much information as possible and doing all the research you can. It may mean changing someone's living environment, changing doctors, changing medication, or trying new techniques. Being proactive is about making a change.

Prepare yourself, as sometimes changing things won't make a difference and you can think "what is the point?" but by making that change it may lead you closer to the right change because it has eliminated one dead end and it can give you peace of mind that it wasn't what you changed that was at fault for something going wrong. I would rather know definite answers than live my life in a world of 'what ifs' and 'could have beens.'

Don't be afraid to tweak things constantly. Being proactive may not just be about big changes but small changes that can make a big difference. Especially when trying something new, you may need to work on it and tweak it to make it work or for it to help. Don't forget, also, that sometimes changes take a little while to take effect so don't be disillusioned if you don't see results on day one. If you believe in what you are doing, try to give it a chance to see if it can work before giving up on it or moving in another direction.

Sometimes making things better involves work and may require you knocking on lots of doors and going down lots of dead ends. Sadly, nobody has knowledge on everything or a crystal ball to predict the future. There is no AA-approved route to get what you need or to make things better. Being proactive is about blazing your own trail, not waiting for things to be given to you or accepting the first answer you hear.

CHAPTER TWENTY-NINE

Nothing Lasts Forever

One thing you have to live with is the knowledge and understanding that nothing lasts forever. Good times don't last forever, easy times don't last forever but the same can be said for bad and hard times, too. You've got to enjoy every day and make the most of it as you never know when things are going to change or when things are going to come to an end. When you are going through bad times it is important to remember that they don't last forever and remember the good times whilst you await their return.

Try where you can to be ready for the changes and when changes do happen you need to be able to accept them. There is no point not accepting change as it goes on regardless of whether you want it to or not. The other thing to remember is that change might be only temporary. There's nothing to say that things will stay that way long term so you have to be ready to roll with it and experience it when it happens.

If you think the good times or the bad times will last forever then you are a fool. When you go through bad times it makes you appreciate how good the good times were and when life gets even worse again you start thinking back to what you thought were bad times and think to yourself that they were actually pretty good. Sometimes you just don't know how good you have got it, and how good you think you have got it depends on your view on life of what is good and what is bad.

I lost my mum too early and I thought my mum would be around forever. I thought we would get longer to care for her but she declined very rapidly. I thought I would dedicate the rest of my life to caring for my mum but that didn't happen. I never thought life would ever be good again but bit by bit it is improving. Never assume, double guess or try to predict the future. There are some changes that will just happen if you want them to and there are some changes you can stop if you want to. Life is about picking when is the right time to let change happen naturally and when you need to fight to make it happen. It's not an exact science and it's not easy but do it well and you will have an amazing life.

Emotions, events, time and life; just a few examples of things that don't last forever. These are things that can seem long whilst you are going through them or about to go through them but looking back can be just like fleeting moments in a rich life full of interesting stories.

CHAPTER THIRTY

Memories

I think it is important to make as many good memories as you possibly can when caring for a loved one. When the time comes that your caring role ends they will be a comfort to look back on. When caring for someone, days can very easily just roll one into another and weeks pass without you really noticing. When you are in the midst of the situation it's hard sometimes to take a step back. You spend all your time prioritising the necessary caring tasks you have to complete that this can take all your energy and can consume all your thoughts.

With my mum I didn't document our life together enough. You can never have too many photos, too many videos, too many pieces of writing, so never miss an opportunity. I wish I had more photos and videos of my mum. Since she passed I have spent a lot of time trying to find as many as possible and to look at them on a regular basis. Photos and videos aren't just good for you; they are good to have to show future generations of the family in years to come and to show them what your loved one was like when they were with us.

I love photo albums. I think photos need to be printed, need to be displayed and need to be shared and not just stored on a computer or a roll of film. Not only the memories they create but also the fun in taking the photos, the fun in finding a frame to display them and the fun in making photo albums is what I enjoy.

Putting photos in frames and photo albums is something in which you can involve your family and the loved one you are caring for. This will help make these photos mean even more and create even more memories to enjoy later in life.

As well as documenting things, try to make as many memories as possible by doing special things for your loved one so you can both have a lovely moment and create that memory that lasts a lifetime. I spent every day trying to create special memories and moments for my mum. Whenever I went shopping I would look for something to get mum that she would like and always thinking of places we could go. I always wanted to make every day different and always wanted to make every situation the best it could be. I would take what some would see as an ordinary daily task or outing and try to make it special and different somehow. At the other level, if we were doing something interesting and cool I would still try to make it even more special and unique.

When doing something with the loved one you are caring for, the more entertaining and happy you can make it for everyone the better. Eventually, when looking back on life, you want to make sure that the number of good memories outweighs the bad. I think if people can remember happy moments, events and days it can help them deal with grief and sadness a lot better. A good memory that brings a smile to the face of the loved one you are caring for is worth more than anything you could ever put a price on and may help them in ways that they will never be able to communicate with you. Life isn't about the number of days you have on this earth, it's about what you do with the days you have.

Treasure memories always; don't be in a rush to discard them. Memories provide great talking points and can stimulate so many thoughts and thought processes. They can take you back to happier times, they can help you remember people and times in your life. Memories can sometimes be a reason to cry and sometimes a reason to smile but we should treasure them in equal measure. When everything else is gone memories are the only thing we have left. Memories are the most important possessions I own as they help me to remember mum always.

I think people should be encouraged to cry, to smile, to laugh. I think it is important to do this to help process and deal with the situation you are going through. Anything that encourages people not to bottle things up is positive in my eyes. Memories are things that encourage people to think about the situation and to feel it emotionally, which is important, especially long-term. I don't think anything or anyone should be forgotten and memories are one of the most important and strongest ways of keeping someone alive in your heart.

My hope in life is that I gave mum a million and one positive memories and that she kept as many as she possibly could right up to the end. Even though her condition robbed her of so many functions and ways of communication, I hope that in her head she saw positive and happy things. Mum has already given me more than a lifetime's worth of happy memories, which will always outweigh the bad no matter how bad I feel. This is one of the greatest things I can say about my mum; that every day we shared was memorable.

CHAPTER THIRTY-ONE

Holiday

As I've already mentioned, one of my fondest memories and one of the proudest things we did was take mum on holiday to Australia in 2011 for three weeks whilst she was still able to fly. It had always been mum's dream to go to Australia and the more days pass, the more proud I am that we got the chance to do it. It is one of the few things about the last five years that I look back on and smile about. Changing the scenery and seeing mum's dreams comes true will always make Australia a happy place for me, where nothing bad existed and only dreams came true.

I would recommend a holiday to any family caring for someone, where the whole family goes, including the loved one you are caring for. Changing the scenery makes everyone happier and that feeling of being on holiday just lets people forget for a moment and let loose. Holidays are places where memories that last a lifetime are made.

It doesn't need to be a big holiday. You don't have to go abroad, just somewhere different from your home environment. A holiday can provide extra challenges for the caring of your loved one but the positives outweigh the negatives for a while and can improve the way you care when you go back home. You will feel more positive, you will have had a good time and you will hopefully be more refreshed than when you went. Holidays break the cycle and take you out of the day-to-day routine, which is such a refreshing feeling. Holidays will hopefully improve your mental, emotional and physical state.

We didn't have the money really to go on the holiday but we found it. We didn't let anything stop us or stand in our way because you can't put a price on making dreams happen. It was the least we could do for a mum who had given us so much and done so much for us.

The weather in Australia was awesome, which was good for my mum as she struggled with cold weather and the people were friendly and went out of their way to help us have an amazing time. It may be cliché but it truly was a holiday of a lifetime. Seeing mum enjoying herself without the cares of the world was the most amazing feeling and three weeks I will never forget.

Going on holiday can present challenges and make it slightly more difficult to perform basic caring duties that you do for your loved one so it is important you research and plan properly before you depart. Make sure you have a supply of everything you need to care for your loved one. Be ready to improvise and be patient when administering care. If you are travelling on public transport like a boat or a plane, inform the staff so they will be able to be sensitive to your situation and help where they can. Leave plenty of time for your journeys to and from places. It's your job to take any possible stress out of the holiday, as there is no point in going if it is just going to stress you out even more.

Don't be afraid to ask someone to come with you to help. The more people you have helping you, the easier it will be on everyone. The person or people helping you can free you up to help your loved one by taking care of getting you between places and dealing with any staff or public situations you may by faced with. They can handle all the checking in and make arrangements on your behalf.

CHAPTER THIRTY-TWO

Legacy

With more and more people having to care for a loved one at some point in their life, surely we should be educating kids about this in school. I think advice and teaching on what to do if called to care for a loved one would be really important life advice that could help so many young people. Children should be taught what to do, how to handle it and who to contact. Doing this would help the care levels for ill people and help the mental and emotional health of the one having to give the care. The care industry is a big employment field in the UK right now so it would also give young people a skill they could use to gain employment.

I think you are very naïve if you don't think you will ever have to care for somebody in some capacity in your lifetime. I think we need to shift people into the mindset that it is just part of normal life and nothing to run away from, be ashamed about or be unduly unnerved by. Once you get people in that mindset then you can start teaching people how to deal with it when it does happen. To get people who aren't currently caring for someone or have no one sick in their life to learn about caring before you have made them realise how much of a real possibility it is won't work.

I think if you educated and prepared people from a young age the stigma around caring would change, society would have more sympathy for people giving care and instead of just moving loved ones into homes or expecting others to pick up the pieces, more family members would be empowered to care for their loved ones. I also think people would then make more allowances for people caring for a loved one and would do more to make their life easier.

Young people are our future and given the right education will go on later in life to think more about caring for others or helping people who do. So if they run a business that deals with the public they might try and make their place more accessible for someone bringing in a loved one they care for. If they become a manager of staff they will be more flexible with staff if they are caring for a loved one. If they got into politics they might choose to do something to help people caring for loved ones. If we educate people early, this world will become a much easier and better place for those caring for others.

All of this would save the government and NHS a lot of money long term in the care and support for people in the country with long-term sickness. It would also save money in supporting people struggling emotionally and with mental ill health following the news of a loved one needing care. It may enable people to say in their jobs for longer and not have to take time off with stress so it would also boost the economy.

Most importantly, by educating people early you will improve the level of care loved ones get when they get diagnosed with long-term illnesses. There is a financial incentive for the government to encourage schools to do work on caring for people with long-term illnesses but I think it would also benefit the level of care and the mental health of the person doing the caring.

An important part of writing this book has been about a legacy for my mum and I would love to be involved and spearhead developments in caring so that I can use my experiences of caring for my mum to help others. I know my mum would have loved to help others going through similar problems that we went through as a family if she were still with us.

We can have all the knowledge we want on a subject but without action it is pretty useless. That is why I am so keen that this book or I personally can help create some real and practical change to help so many people going through similar situations. This is one way I can see it being possible. If we help people who are currently caring for loved ones and prepare the ones who may at some point in their life have to become carers then this world will be in a pretty good state to deal with this ever-growing issue.

CHAPTER THIRTY-THREE

Why Did I Write This Book?

I wrote this book to keep a promise I made to my mum. But the reason I offered to write this for mum was because I wanted to help and do something positive, do something that might just change a life, a country, a world. Too many people think they don't know enough to share or that their experience isn't worth sharing. I think as a nation in Britain, on the whole, we are very modest and private people but I think this gets in our way at times of really coming together and making a bit of change.

There are lots of taboos that you don't think you are allowed to talk about or don't feel right bringing up in conversation. That is the great thing about writing this book as it has given me the ability to write about emotions, feelings and events that I wouldn't have the strength or the bravery to talk about in public.

The level of care someone gets now seems to be determined by the area they live in, the family they are born into and the money they have. I don't want to live in a world like this and I hate that even with an NHS free health system this is still the case. Everyone suffering from the same problem should get the same level of care, no matter what circumstances they find themselves in. I can't change the NHS by myself but I can hope that this book gets widely read and that it inspires people and that people share the information in this book.

Everyone has their own way they can help and make a difference and I think this book is mine. It may not be the best written book in the world but I hope that through it I have been able to convey my passion and share valuable knowledge and experience that will help those who read it. If someone gets helped by just one piece of advice, one chapter, one sentence, one word, one feeling, then this process will have been extremely worthwhile. The most important and best things in life aren't always easy to achieve so let's get out there and try to help as many people achieve them as possible.

Words, books, writing now in the modern age can get everywhere thanks to the online world so I think more than ever it is a good time to get information out there. Writing is no longer confined to a paper book that you have to go to a shop to buy or a library to borrow. I hope to bring this book out in as many formats as possible, as I really believe now more than ever that words can change the world.

CHAPTER THIRTY-FOUR

One Year On

So it's one year on from when my mum passed and I am finally coming to the end of writing this book. I have found it an interesting six months, with lots of ups and downs. When your life is so much about one person for so long and then they aren't there any more it is very hard to readjust. Daily routines and priorities change overnight and reasons for living have to change with it.

My main purpose behind writing this book was to share my story and the information I gained just in case it helped just one person and if I manage to do that with this book then it will be a way of keeping my mum's legacy going. I promised my mum before she passed that I would write a book so I am glad to have kept that promise. Writing the book gave me something to focus on in the hard days and weeks after my mum passed. It gave me space to talk about how I felt and process the experiences and the emotions of the last four years. It helped me find reasons why certain things happened and why I felt certain things in certain ways.

I'm glad I got on with writing the book very quickly after mum passed. Some may say it was too quick and that I needed time to heal but I just didn't want any of my memories or feelings to fade away or become less strong or less clear. I wanted every emotion and feeling as raw and fresh as it could be. I know also the longer I left it to start the harder it would become and there was less of a chance of me actually getting on with it. To break a promise to my mum would have been heartbreaking.

I just hope mum would have liked this book and that it is what my mum would have wanted. I hope that the book is honouring to her memory and that it will help more people remember my mum or get to know who my mum was and why she was so special to me. I wish the world could have known about my mum when she was alive but the best I can do now is share how amazing I thought she was.

Who knows what the next six months, six years or six decades will hold? I will continue to take mum with me in my heart wherever I go and just see where life takes me. I know she would have wanted the best for me, like I wanted the best for her. I just hope that with this book and with my life that I made you proud, mum, as that was and is all I ever want to do.

When somebody dies, for everyone else life goes on. You may want it to stop for a while or you may not feel like going on but the world and people around you don't stop. It is important to mourn and we should all take time to do that but my philosophy is "why waste a day that the person who died would have loved to have?" I bet the person who died wouldn't want you to waste your days or stop living; they would want you to make the best of the opportunities you have. There isn't any shame or blame in wanting to get on with life and make the most of every day.

It may not seem like it after someone has died but every day is a blessing and should be treated as such. Go out and live it the fullest you can. To me, the best way of honouring and appreciating someone's life is to go out and make the most of yours. I want to continue to show the world that my mum was an excellent mum and it was because of the way she raised me that I am now able to make a good contribution to this world and I can let everyone know that this is all because of my mum. I can keep her legacy going and honour her in my words and my actions every day. If I stay being miserable then that's not a very good honouring of my mum's skills in raising me and if I stay inside and never go out then nobody else will ever have the chance to hear about or find out about my mum. By me going out and being around people it also helps others as it gives them the chance to talk about and think about my mum and I know my mum loved the fact that I spent so much time helping others, as that is exactly what she spent her time doing.

An important thing to do is never to judge anybody about the way they live their life after a death. Different people handle it in different ways and unless you are in their shoes you don't know what they are going through. The important thing is to love and support them the best you can. On the judging front, don't judge yourself either for what you are doing and the way you are handling things. Judging yourself will only lead to more distress, sadness and depression. Don't hide away from emotions and feelings; give yourself space and time to be yourself.

Try to not push others away in the wake of the death of a loved one. It is very easy to push people away but it's important not to as one day you may need them. If they are a good person and know you well they will understand that you are only doing it because of the way you are feeling at that time and will stick around, but not everyone will so be very careful.

After caring for someone so long it may be a pattern you fall into and you just move on to caring for someone else. It may be in a different way, like looking out for someone else in the family who is grieving, but it is still taking on that caring role. Or you might want to go and help someone who is going through the same as what your loved one went through. Just remember that you don't have to do it and it is OK to take a break from being that person, as it is not the only thing you are. I'm not saying don't do it if you want to but just don't think you have to and that caring is all you are good at. Try to remember what you did before you started caring for your loved one and what you enjoyed doing.

There is no saying you will want to do those things or enjoy doing those things now but you don't know until you try.

CHAPTER THIRTY-FIVE

My Mum

My mum wasn't just my mum – she was also my best friend and my biggest supporter.

Every morning mum would get us up and make us breakfast. She would then give us our lunch that she had made and wave us off. Mum would then be there to pick us up from school at the end of the day, make us dinner and then help us with anything we needed. At weekends she would give up her Saturdays to take me around Cornwall and Devon for football, which would sometimes mean two or three games, starting early and getting home late.

The illness robbed mum of so much but it never took her amazing spirit, personality and character, which filled any room she was in, and she did this without words but by her presence alone. My mum was a person you would never forget, even if you just met her once. Mum fought her illness with great bravery, courage and dignity. She never took the easy way out and faced it head on.

Mum's life should not be defined by her illness but by the amazing impact she had on all who knew her. She was an incredible mum to me, David and Mark. Mum dedicated herself to giving us the best life possible, not spending a penny or a second on herself. Nothing was too much to ask for mum. If we wanted something she would find a way of making it happen. She would drive us anywhere we wanted to go, fight our battles for us, support us in anything we wanted to do and kept the house up straight so we could just concentrate on being kids.

I just hope that one day I can be half as good a parent as my mum was, as to me being a parent is one of the most important jobs anyone can be entrusted with and mum was the best at it.

My goal in life has been to make mum's life as enjoyable as possible, even more so over the last three years, and it is that mission that has given me my drive and my reason to get up every day and face the world. But now mum isn't with us in person I can't continue that mission. Instead, I will get a new one: to make sure nobody forgets you, mum, to continue your legacy and to make you proud every day I have on this earth until one day I am with you again.

Mum, you made me who I am and I just hope I can make you as proud of me as I am of you.

What I said at my mum's funeral 24/01/13.

CHAPTER THIRTY-SIX

Family

I don't think I can write this book without dedicating a chapter to my family. Each one of them individually has helped me so much and made our family what it is. Without my family we would not have been able to give mum the level of care she got and be inspired to keep fighting every day for her. All my family over the last few years have made amazing sacrifices and endured the harshest of pains and I am so proud of them.

My dad shouldered the brunt of the responsibility and was hurt the most. My dad was loving and caring to the end and no matter how bad, sad or frustrated he felt still kept soldiering on to the very end. I think when you watch someone care for their partner who is ill you see a whole new level of compassion and love. My dad suffered the most of all of us and suffered most after mum's passing but I am so proud of the way he handled himself throughout the process, never gave up and did the best he possibly could.

When a situation like a parent suffering with dementia happens you see the true test of the family unit, the relationships within the family and the people within it. Nothing can prepare you for it but through it I think it brought out the best of us and made our family stronger. It gives you a reason to keep in touch more and to see each other more if you live far apart. It makes you think of others before yourself and be nicer to members of your family.

Through what happened with my mum it gave me a new level of appreciation of everyone in my family individually and an appreciation of the roles they play in the family. In every family everyone has a part to play and it is what they do and the role they play that can have a big impact on the rest of the unit. In situations like these you can't do it all yourself, you need to be able to rely on those around you to pull their weight and step up to the plate.

My mum loved each and every one of us in the family and it was important for her that she was shown love by everyone and knew she was loved by everyone, which she was. I don't think it is wise in families to see people and roles as more important than each other or to think who your loved one loves more. People will love others in different ways and it is important that you let this happen naturally and never start thinking who loves who more as that is when the family unit breaks down. Every ounce of love in a family is needed so make sure every little bit is expressed and used.

Don't forget when caring for someone in your family it's not just about caring about that person as the more you care for others as well who aren't going through problems the more they will be able to care for your loved one. No care is wasted and all of it is important.

Everyone in your family will handle the situation in different ways and everyone will be affected differently. So don't judge or pre-judge anything or anyone. Give everyone the space and right to handle things in their own way and be there for them always. Never close yourself off from others or give them reason to feel closed off.

So in conclusion remember, when it comes to your family, love everyone, don't expect anything and be there for everyone.

CHAPTER THIRTY-SEVEN

My New Family

I was so lucky that near the end of my mum's time on earth the love of my life walked into my life. My wife and my soul mate, she gave me something outside of the bubble I was living in, she gave me reason to smile, to not give up and a hope of a better life. Jenni supported me throughout, took my mind off the horrible things and let me talk if I wanted to. She was very understanding of my situation, more than anyone else ever would be, and had to be very patient at the beginning –and I mean *very* patient! She had to make sacrifices and build our relationship around me, my mum and my family.

If it were not for Jenni's love and patience we wouldn't have the amazing relationship and life we have now. I will be forever thankful and never be able to repay all the hard work and sacrifice she put in at the beginning. It was hard at the time to balance everything but looking back on it now it was the perfect time and helped me deal with the transition that has been my life in the last few years.

I never had a relationship that my mum knew about but I know that if she could see me now she would be so happy that I am married and so happy that I have found an amazing wife in Jenni. I know she would have loved her. My only unhappiness about the situation is that they never met as they are both amazing people and that mum was not able to be at my wedding. I wish I had been able to give her grandchildren whilst she was still with us on earth. I also wish my mum had been there to see our first house and come to visit for tea and cake all the time. The one thing I will do, though, is to make sure that any of my future children will always know who their grandmother was.

Jenni gives me the strength and courage to continue my work, research and support of those going through similar situations that I experienced and that my family experienced. I can't imagine how hard the time since my mum's passing would have been without her and I will never be able to thank her enough for helping me through it. Because of Jenni, the future looks bright and because of her I am able to look back with more happy memories than sad ones.

Word of Thanks

This book is dedicated to my mum, June Sophia Sibley, who sadly passed away in January 2013.

Thanks go to my amazing family old and new who have been an amazing support, not only through this book-writing process, which has been a tough and hard road, but also for all the way through the roller coaster ride that has been our family life. The last three years could have broken most families and, although we aren't all here any more, I am so proud and glad that our family has not fallen apart and has remained strong for each other throughout the hardest of times.

I can't thank enough my friends who stood by me and never left me; the ones who showed me understanding and supported me; the ones who were patient with me and didn't expect anything in return; the ones who helped me practically and emotionally, as well as the ones who helped me and did things for me that I never found out about. Without these people I would not be where I am today.

I would like to thank my employers, who have been brilliant with me and my situation over recent years. Without their continued employment and their flexibility there would have been many chapters in this book that I wouldn't have been able to write. In a tough economic situation and a fierce job market, I am so thankful I got to keep my job throughout this time and now still have a job today.

I would like to take time to thank the volunteer organisations I help out with: for them taking the burden and load from me in recent years, for not expecting too much from me during this period, for not getting annoyed when I couldn't commit to doing as much as usual and for keeping my position open for me throughout the hardest of times.

I would also like to thank all of mum's carers, doctors and supporters. I know so many people worked so hard to help us keep mum at home for as long as we did. They provided great practical and emotional support for the entire family and came in at a time when we really needed them. I dread to think what the last year would have been like without them. When dealing with these people, although it was their job and what they were paid to do, I got a real sense that they cared and wanted to help, which meant a lot to me.

Lastly, thanks also go to the hundreds of people whose names I don't even know who mum and I came across over the years who went out of their way to help us and our situation. I will never know all your names but I do remember the faces and the way I was touched by all your acts of kindness.

Bad things have happened in life and I have been tested to my limits but I am so thankful for the life I was given and so thankful for the chance to share my thoughts, emotions and experiences through this book. One thing life has taught me recently is be thankful for what you have today as you may not have it tomorrow.

I hope through this book and through my life I can thank my mum for all she ever did for me and, even after her passing, everything she is still doing for me today. Remember never to be afraid to give or say thanks. Never underestimate the power of saying thank you.

Printed in November 2022
by Rotomail Italia S.p.A., Vignate (MI) - Italy